VEGANIST

VEGANIST

LOSE WEIGHT, GET HEALTHY, CHANGE THE WORLD

Kathy Freston

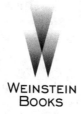

WEINSTEIN
BOOKS

ISBN 978-1-60286-133-6

First Edition
10 9 8 7 6 5 4

Contents

Introduction:
The Big Picture

FIRST OF ALL, LET ME TELL YOU RIGHT OFF THE BAT THAT THIS book is all about the lean—leaning in to a shift in whatever way or whatever pace feels right to you. It's about checking out some new information that could change your life, and then pushing yourself ever so gently in the direction of health. It's not about making a radical conversion. It's not about strict discipline. It's more about empowering you to take your health into your hands in a practical and easy way, while at the same time arousing a broad spiritual awakening. Making profound changes in your life is never a straight path, and it shouldn't be; it's a gradual awakening with lots of twists and turns that happens in its own time. I am hoping that by providing you with ten life-changing promises fulfilled by *moving toward* a plant-based diet, you will find that that awakening time is at hand now (or soon!).

You don't have to do anything at all upon hearing these promises. You can just sit with them, knowing that if you are ever ready for or desirous of change, there is a way to get there. Or you can just nudge yourself a little, and make small changes in what you eat, so that you gradually build a momentum of healthy choices. Either way, the information in this book will open your eyes in a way you may never have considered.

The most exciting thing is that so much is possible. So much is within our power to make better. We can be healthy and happy. And we can do it so easily, simply by adjusting and tweaking our favorite meals so that they are healthier versions of the things we love. Still delicious, still hearty and satisfying. Just healthier. I promise.

Let me tell you a little about me, first of all, so you don't think that I came out of the womb a veganist. I was born in the South and grew up on chicken-fried steak and cheesy grits. I loved nothing more than a vanilla milkshake and barbecue ribs. I had an appetite for meat like anyone else, and I didn't think twice about it. I wasn't a thoughtless person; I was just enjoying my life and eating what tasted good and what I was told was good for me. It wasn't until I was in my thirties that I started considering where my food came from. When I made the shift to being vegetarian, it was gradual. I gave up eating one animal at a time. I'd come home and tell my husband, "I'm not cooking any more steak." He'd roll his eyes and say, "Whatever." And some months later, I'd be standing in the kitchen saying, "I can't put chicken on the table anymore"—he was a little more perturbed about that. Later still, when I said I couldn't bring myself to buy cheese anymore, he thought I'd lost my mind. Luckily, by then, I began hitting my stride with this lean toward a plant-based diet. I found so, so many delicious foods that were actually the same as our favorite meals, but without the meat. Sometimes I brought home meat alternatives (vegetarian versions of chicken or ribs, etc.) and sometimes I focused more on beans, legumes, and whole grains (like black bean burritos with guacamole or lentil soup with cheesy bread and salad).

I actually began to love this food, and so did my husband. He told me, "If I thought I could have eaten this well as a vegetarian, I would have gone that way a long time ago." There was no loss. No stringent diet or "bird food." We simply lightened up on the animal-based foods and replaced them with plant-based fare. Before too long (it was a period of a few years, actually), we had a vegan home and were entertaining friends and family with unbelievably delicious (and nutritious) food.

Mind you, my husband is still not vegan . . . not even vegetarian (although he is certainly leaning in that direction). I am, though, and in our home we have only vegan food. I'm flexible with him (I don't bug him when he orders fish at a restaurant) and he lets me be me. Some of our friends and family have changed their diet because they love the food and see what a difference it's made in me, and some of our friends simply find it interesting cuisine for the time spent at our house. In all cases, I've been thrilled to see how people have gravitated toward and been interested in hearing more. Hence the book!

I want to shine a bright light on the whole world of positives that flow from the decision to eat a plant-based diet—positives for your health (eliminating meat leads naturally, even effortlessly, to weight loss; blood sugar balancing;

prevention, even reversal of heart disease; etc., etc., etc.) but also for your mind and your spirit, positives in terms of feeding the world and keeping the earth from deeper peril, in terms of putting money in your pocket and saving precious natural resources and deepening your sense of kinship with life.

You see, following a vegan (or vegan-ish) diet is a choice that has no downside. It's a home run, a good-for-everyone-and-everything solution. It can help you lose weight, heal your body from disease, *and* start making the world a more peaceful and livable place. And it's as delicious and inexpensive as it is good for our planet Earth.

In an effort to find a word to describe this magnificent tapestry of good that surrounds the choice to eat only food that grows on trees or from the ground, I landed on the term *veganist*. (Actually, my husband, after listening to enough of my spiels, said, "Honey, you're a veganist!" and it stuck.) I intend it as a soft word, a forgiving word. It's not about hard lines or purity or perfection but about intention and holding ideas loosely and taking steps in the direction of the kind of person you want to be, leading the kind of life you want to lead.

Okay, you say, but why would you want to call yourself a veganist? Doesn't that sound like something negative, like a racist or a sexist? No, no, and no! Just like the words "altruist" or "chemist" or "artist," a "veganist" is someone who is intensely interested in a subject and wants to go on learning more. The suffix "-ist" means "one who does." Veganists take action on what they learn—not necessarily in an "activist" way but in whatever works to make their individual lives better while perhaps also helping to make the world a better place.

The "-ist" also refers to "one who studies." A veganist is one who looks closely at all the implications of his or her food choices—to his or her own body, to the animals and the land it takes to raise them and the drugs introduced to keep herds alive, and so on, and then decides how to act. I like the idea of upgrading an old word that had some off-putting connotations; for many the word *vegan* calls to mind dogmatic hippies who eat nothing but granola and sprouts. No thanks on that. What I'm talking about are people who don't mix up being passionate about getting healthy and happy with self-deprivation, and whose radiant well-being shows in everything they do.

Eating a diet of whole grains, beans, vegetables, and fruits, along with meat alternatives like veggie burgers or "chick'n" patties or soy dogs thrown in, your body will change on so many levels. Your metabolism will straighten out, enabling you to lose weight, if you need to, in a slow, steady, sustainable way. You will no longer feel led around by the mood swings and cravings that fatty and processed foods can cause; your skin will clear up and take on a permanent glow; your circulation (and with it your capacity for sexual pleasure!) will improve; and as study after study has been showing, you dramatically reduce your chances of getting heart disease, stroke, and diabetes and quite possibly cancer.

As if these weren't reasons enough, according to reputable scientists like Cornell nutrition professor T. Colin Campbell, PhD, and the Cleveland Clinic's Caldwell Esselstyn, MD, among others, you can even *halt and reverse* many diseases when you embrace a plant-based diet. There is a must-see film out called *Forks over Knives* (*forksoverknives .com*), which is a documentary about the work of these two amazing researchers. You'll hear from them in this book, and also from other leading medical experts on diet and health. You will also find first-person accounts of people who overcame life-threatening and debilitating diseases through their shift to a plant-based diet.

But the personal health benefits are just one part of the story, albeit a very important one. What about the social and environmental benefits I mentioned above? It seems clearer every day that the planet thrives for every person who chooses to eat more plant-based fare, because animal agriculture is one of the top culprits in creating a host of very serious environmental problems. You've undoubtedly read other books or seen movies, newspaper articles, or blogs detailing the horrors of animal slaughter and meat "processing." But, you see, here's one area of our lives where we actually have some control. We can simply say, "No thanks; I'll take the vegetarian option!" and stop participating in something that feels wrong.

This will be a bit of an adjustment, but going easy with yourself and leaning in will help enormously. Remember, all you have to do is take in the information, and lean toward better choices. Gradually. At your own pace. You can choose nondairy milks that, frankly, taste better than regular old milk. You can replace your beloved BLT and have tempeh (vegetarian) bacon on your sandwich instead. It's really so much fun to find foods that are simply upgraded versions of the ones you grew up loving.

Maybe you've heard that eating vegan will help you lose weight. Maybe it's your affection for animals that's driving you to take a look at your diet. Or maybe you read somewhere that it takes sixteen pounds of grain to produce one pound of meat and realized that if you stopped eating meat you might help feed the world. Any of these would be reason enough to reduce your meat consumption. But once you do that you find all the other benefits too.

Being a veganist is good for your health, it's good for the environment, and it's certainly good for the animals, but it also has a powerful spiritual component. When you begin eating consciously, with compassion and thoughtfulness, you attain a certain lightness and inner peace, a sense of connectedness to the larger world. When you lean more toward a plant-based diet, you help liberate acres of farmland to grow food for more humans, not more pent-up cows and pigs and chickens. And that also connects you to the web of life. It's all upside.

It feels so good and empowering to know that we are bigger than our habits and hankerings, that we can actually make a subtle switch in what we put on our plates for the promise of a better life all around. It feels so liberating to know that we can be in charge of our well-being and our choices, and that those choices will ripple out in their effects, both personally and globally.

That's what this is about too. Being a veganist (or veganish) is about choosing behaviors that support your values, that make a positive contribution to the kind of world you want to live in. Our food choices can contribute directly to well-being and consciousness, or they can do just the oppo-site. It's so completely up to us.

How to Read This Book

The book is organized into ten promises and is packed with information, some of which will appeal to you right now and some of which might just be too much to take during the first read. I know, because it took me years to get around to read-ing certain books; I avoided delving into the truth about how what we eat affects us and the world around us, because much of it was simply a shock to my system and made me really uncomfortable. I recommend that you browse the table of contents and then start with the chapters that appeal to you and circle back to the others when you are ready to layer on some more information. For instance, you may be in-terested in weight loss and cancer prevention, but don't really want to look at animal cruelty right now. Or you might want to take a good look at the spiritual aspect of diet and also understand about how the food industry affects the global food supply. Personally, my favorite chapters are the last two (Promises 9 and 10) because I tend to be more inter-ested in spirituality and personal growth. And the Afterword is practically a whole book in itself because it's chock-full of tips and information on how to make changes of habit, so definitely read that. But I completely understand if the mid-dle of the book becomes overwhelming; it *is* a lot of infor-mation. Feel free to skip around, dipping in and out of the subjects that catch your attention; the information will surely trickle in. If you encounter something that makes you un-comfortable, please don't put the book down or stop reading;

just move on to the chapters that are most compelling to you. Then lean in a little more when you're ready and inform yourself at a pace that's comfortable for you. There is some fascinating information within these pages, and I expect you will want to digest it according to the pace that feels right to you.

No matter where you are on this journey—whether you have cut back on eating meat already or are just starting to consider what that might look like—get ready for some miracles. Truly. Taking animals out of your diet is a game changer.

VEGANIST

Promise 1:

Your Body Will Find and Maintain Its Ideal Weight—Effortlessly

Did you know?

- On a healthful vegan diet, weight comes off effortlessly and sustainably, without calorie counting.
- Fiber, which is only found in plant-based foods, is something of a weight-loss magician. It fills your stomach quickly (by holding water) and fools your brain into thinking you are full.
- A plant-based diet revs your metabolism, causing you to burn calories up to 16% faster than you would on a non-plant-based diet for at least the first 3 hours after meals.
- Most of us only overeat when we're eating the wrong foods. When we're eating healthfully, our bodies know when to stop and "turn off" our hunger switch.

- Plant-based foods are naturally low in fat. It's very hard to be—or stay—overweight on a vegan diet.

- A fat gram has 9 calories; a carbohydrate has only 4. By avoiding fats—like these found in meat and cheese—you avoid lots of calories.

- The quick results some people get with high-animal protein, low-carb diets don't last because most of the loss is water—or unsustainable calorie deprivation.

- It's simply a myth that vegans have a hard time getting enough protein. Besides, most Americans eat far more protein than their bodies need or can successfully use. And because it comes from animals, the protein is accompanied by a lot of fat, too.

- Processed carbohydrates like the ones found in white bread, conventional cakes and cookies, and your basic junk food give you a cheap high and a fast crash, causing you to keep eating. The carbs found in whole grains give you energy over a much longer period of time and spare you the crash (and subsequent binge) altogether.

Anyone who has struggled with weight knows how hard it can be to lose it and especially to keep it off. Even those of us who aren't seriously overweight often struggle with extra pounds that we're just not comfortable with, or find ourselves embarrassed by a body image we instinctively know is not right.

There are probably a thousand different programs and diets out there promising quick weight loss, and most dieters will try several over the course of a lifetime—with only limited success. As you've no doubt heard or read or experienced, most dieters end up losing and gaining back hundreds of pounds over a lifetime, and usually gain back more than they've lost in each successive round. Why? To put it very simply, it's because with all these big dietary shifts the metabolism gets really confused and can't settle on "normal." When you eat a mostly plant-based diet, all that changes.

Eating vegan is not a weight-loss program per se, but weight loss *is* one of the great side effects of eating a healthy, plant-based diet. But you don't have to take it just from me. Later in this chapter you'll be able to listen in on my conversation with Dr. Dean Ornish, who probably knows more about the way fats are processed in our bodies than anyone on the planet. He will explain, in easy-to-understand terms, just why our bodies process food so efficiently when we stop eating animals or at least move toward a plant-based diet.

A moment of truth here: If you continue to eat processed foods full of sugar and fat, you won't lose weight. But you knew that. And that's not why you're here. You're here to discover how good you'll feel on a diet of vegetarian proteins, whole grains, and all the glorious and diverse vegetables and fruits of the earth.

If you look around, you won't see many fat vegans. Vegans tend to be slim and strong, gorgeous and glowing, and that's because a healthy, plant-based diet creates vitality and vigor—and weight loss simply happens as a result of not eating fatty animal protein.

And lest you think a plant-based diet is for weaklings, consider bulls, elephants, gorillas, orangutans, and stallions. These plant eaters are pure lean and powerful muscle.

Of course some people think vegans are thin because once you eliminate meat there's nothing good left to eat or because we're unbearably choosy eaters. Hardly! When you start focusing your diet on plant-based foods, a magnificent array of flavors and colors and textures and aromas opens to you and awakens your appetite to some really incredible vegetarian dishes.

We've become so accustomed to the taste of salt and sugar and the mouthfeel of fats, but once we move toward this other way of eating, we find that we lose our taste for thick, greasy, and unhealthy foods and that eating nonanimal foods leaves us feeling light and energized.

The Diet Your Body Is Designed For

The fact is our bodies aren't meant to ingest meat and dairy and eggs and fish. That's right, our bodies aren't meant to eat animals; they're made for whole grains, vegetarian proteins like beans and legumes, fruits and vegetables, nuts and seeds. We may be omnivores in that our bodies are *capable* of living on just about anything—flesh included—in times of scarcity. But unless you are living in sub-Saharan Africa or some isolated part of the North Pole, scarcity is, fortunately, not a problem. In fact we are blessed with abundance. Our modern problem is obesity and all the degenerative diseases that are linked to obesity, like cancer, heart disease, and type 2 diabetes.

When we eat what our bodies were designed for, we thrive. All we have to do is look at what our own physiology shows us: Our molars are like those of an herbivore, flat and blunt, making them good for grinding, not gnashing and tear-ing. Our hands are nimble and flexible and great for picking fruits from trees and scooping vegetables from the ground; they don't have claws to tear open flesh. We don't have the concentration of hydrochloric acid in our stomachs necessary for the proper digestion of raw meat. And finally, a carnivore's intestine is short and straight—perfect for quickly getting rid of rotting flesh, whereas ours is long and winding with notches along the inside that slow down the digestive process. Meat often rots on its way through our complex digestive system. There is an excellent article that covers all these details and more, titled "The Comparative Anatomy of Eating," by Dr. Milton Mills, which you can easily find online.

When the American Dietetic Association (ADA) surveyed all the studies on food and health, they concluded not just that a vegetarian or vegan diet is as healthy as one that includes meat, but that "vegetarians have been reported to have lower body mass indices than non-vegetarians, as well as lower rates of death from ischemic heart disease, lower blood cholesterol levels, lower blood pressure, and lower rates of hypertension, type 2 diabetes, and prostate and colon cancer."

Among the many diets that have been popular over the past few decades, probably few have been more influential—or controversial—than carbohydrate-elimination diets. Yes, they promise—and often deliver—quick and substantial weight loss, but sadly most of them seem to be unsustainable and unhealthy, not to mention unscientific. Not only do they not work over the long run, but with their emphasis on animal foods, they're making us fatter ultimately, while at the same time they are likely creating profound problems with our health. They make reassuring promises that we can keep eating the things we love—like cheeseburgers, chicken wings, bacon, turkey sausage, and the like—as long as we avoid the demonized carbohydrates. These trendy diets cause us great harm in so many ways.

For starters, they have people eating quantities of animal protein that our bodies simply cannot handle. As a culture we are eating twice as much animal protein as we did in the early part of the twentieth century. At the same time we have grown dangerously overweight, with more life-challenging illnesses plaguing our health-care system than at any other time in history. As I write this, three out of every five Americans is considered overweight or obese, and two out of every three of us will die of a disease that is strongly linked to obesity. And despite the fact that so much attention has been paid to this issue, as a nation our kids are getting more and more obese with each passing year. We should be alarmed by this and looking for every alternative.

The body recognizes when it has good nutrition and "turns off" the hunger switch because it has what it needs. On the other hand, when you eat heavy, fatty foods you get "addicted" to the richness and need ever more to feel satisfied. Thus, the cycle of overeating kicks in, and you never really feel fulfilled.

Your body is an amazing machine; it's constantly calculating what's coming in through the food you ingest, and it registers whether you are getting enough calories and nutrients to satisfy your needs. To help with this process, there are receptors in your digestive tract which notify your brain how much and what kind of nutrients and calories are being processed. A sort of switch goes off when we are satiated, and we therefore stop eating. That's how nature intended it. But with massive advertising campaigns glorifying fast food and steak dinners and making it all look so tasty and fun to eat, it's no wonder we start craving—and going for—that sort of heavy, fatty food. When we indulge, those natural-born internal receptors get thrown off. The unnaturally high amount of concentrated calories throws the system off, which leads to overeating.

No matter how many calories you are ingesting, if you aren't getting what you need nutritionally, your body sends you out for more in the form of cravings or a yearning to eat something else. It's a primal urge, and hard to ignore. It's literally a survival mechanism that kicks in.

The body is saying (sometimes rather urgently), "I haven't gotten enough nutrients, go get more food!" The problem is that meat, cheese, and refined carbs don't have what it takes to satisfy the body's needs, so the body is never satiated on a diet that is made up mostly of animal protein and junky processed food. In order to truly feel fulfilled, you need to eat good nutrient-dense, fiber-rich food. When you do, your body will feel filled up (the stretch receptors will say, "Ah, enough, thank you!"), and because you will have satisfied your essential need for real nutrients, your body will leave you alone. You will not be assailed by constant, gnawing cravings, and in essence, your hunger will be turned off. A general lack of nutrition is one of the main causes of overeating, but when you consume whole, natural foods full of fiber and vitamins, the tendency to overeat goes away and you naturally settle in to your optimal weight. You can read more about this in an excellent book called *The Pleasure Trap* by Douglas J. Lisle, PhD, and Alan Goldhamer, DC.

So why have these high-protein, low-carbohydrate diets (think Atkins, the Zone, and Eat Right for Your Blood Type) stayed around for so long? Probably because most of us have developed a great love for the taste of rich, fatty food and gratefully follow the advice of anyone who says it's okay to keep eating it. Simple as that, really; we want to be told it's okay (and good!) to keep doing what we're doing. But alas, high animal protein with low carbs is *not* a good idea. Not at all. Kathleen Zelman, a spokesperson from the American Dietetic Association, in fact, calls Atkins "a nightmare diet." And a study published in the *Journal of the American Dietetic Association* found that people who were on the diet for only twelve weeks experienced substantially heightened levels of "bad" (LDL) cholesterol. The effects differ from one person to the next, but for some the problems persist, which points to a much higher risk for heart attacks.

Dr. Neal Barnard, founder of the Physician's Committee for Responsible Medicine (PCRM) explains the problem this way:

> Low-carb diets are based on the mistaken notion that bread, potatoes, rice, and beans are fattening, and so these foods are banished from the diet. When you stop eating carbohydrates, your body rapidly loses water. In the first

few days of a low-carb diet, you'll be in the bathroom surprisingly often, and the first few pounds of "weight loss," are not fat loss at all. They are temporary water loss. That water weight will soon come back.

Over the longer period, a low-carb diet causes weight loss only because carbohydrates are about half of what most people eat. If you take away all the pasta, fruit, bread, potatoes, and other carbohydrate-rich foods, you are taking away half of your normal diet. Now, if you make up for it with an equal amount of high-protein and high-fat foods, your weight loss will grind to a halt. Low-carb dieters soon discover that they'll only lose weight when the amount of carbohydrate-rich foods they cut out of their diet is greater than the amount of high-protein, high-fat foods that take their place.

The biggest problem with low-carbohydrate diets is that they teach you a lie. They tell you that high-fat eating is healthy eating. They take you away from healthy fruits and vegetables, and make you feel guilty for eating rice or pasta. Not surprisingly, many people on these diets find that their cholesterol levels skyrocket. Not only do the lost pounds return, but your health can suffer as well.

So basically, the high–animal protein, low-carb diet appears to work at first because of water loss (this happens because the body, starving for glucose normally found in carbs, is using up stored glycogen, which holds a lot of water— 1 pound glycogen holds 3 pounds of water; the first bit of weight loss you see on the low-carb diet is just water loss from losing your natural glycogen, and as soon as you allow a few carbs back in, your water weight comes right back). The diet keeps working for a bit simply because you are cutting out so many of the things you used to eat—you're cutting calories. It will eventually cease working and could cause you serious health problems. The problem is that most people can only keep up the rigid carbohydrate restriction for so long, and even Atkins relaxes the restriction as the diet proceeds to its maintenance phase. As they bring back the range of foods they were eating before, their calorie intake rises back to where it had been. This losing and gaining is, of course, incredibly disheartening but also very unhealthy.

What to Eat to Lose Weight without Going Hungry

Eat fiber rich food! Fiber not only reduces cholesterol and keeps you regular, but it also fools your brain into thinking you are full. It holds water so your stomach feels full. You won't go overboard with too many calories because you feel satisfied—thus, no weight gain. And fiber is only found in plant-based foods like whole grains, beans, veggies, and fruits.

Another mechanism underlying the craving and overeating cycle is blood sugar and insulin imbalance. When we feed our bodies nutrient-dense, fiber-rich, whole foods, which are absorbed slowly and steadily, the craving-overeating cycle is again broken. Whole grains like brown rice, steel-cut oatmeal, and quinoa are ideal staples that will keep you feeling full and satisfied. When grains are processed, however, like the flour used in white bread and the white rice served in most restaurants, the fiber so necessary for the proper *slow* processing and digestion of food and the release of a steady supply of energy is stripped out, along with many other vital nutrients. The refined carbohydrates that are left (you know, the ones you get from most pastries, breads, and cereals) are released almost immediately into the bloodstream. Our bodies read these refined carbohydrates sort of like they do sugar, and we get a quick high followed by a crash, followed by a craving for another hit. When we say we're addicted to cookies or chips, we're not entirely wrong.

Unrefined complex carbohydrates from whole grains like brown rice or kasha (buckwheat groats), yams or sweet potatoes, lentils or chickpeas, on the other hand, are very important for healthy weight and should be a central part of your diet. They break down slowly during digestion and provide the body and brain with a steady and gradual source of energy.

This is where the low-carb brainwashing we've all been fed really led us wrong. We may not need white bread, but we do need unrefined carbohydrates from whole foods! Don't drive yourself too crazy trying to be perfect. Just try to stick to foods that are still in their natural state, unrefined and unprocessed, and you'll find the weight simply melting off.

As Dr. Barnard advises: the key is to think about which carbohydrate foods are best.

Refined carbs give us a cheap high and a fast crash, like sugar or drugs. Whole-food carbs, by contrast, deliver a slow, even dose of energy, keeping us feeling fuller longer.

Here's a handy guide from PCRM:

Instead of sugar, have fruit. Yes, fruit is sweet, but it has little effect on blood sugar.

Instead of white breads, favor rye or pumpernickel. Yes, even whole wheat can cause problems of inflammation.

Instead of white baking potatoes, have yams and sweet potatoes.

Instead of typical cold cereals, have steel-cut oatmeal (the long-cooking kind) or bran cereal. Rice and pasta are fine. Although whole grain pastas are best, even white pasta has a low glycemic index. But make sure you skip the meat and cream sauces and stick to a low-fat tomato sauce.

Meat alternatives are also okay. They are naturally lower in fat and calories and, because they look and taste like the foods we grew up with—bacon, chicken, hot dogs—they can help wean you off meat.

And how about this interesting tidbit from Dr. Barnard: meat stimulates insulin release. Whereas it is common knowledge that refined carbohydrates cause the body to release a lot of insulin, recent studies show that meat also causes a "distinct, sometimes surprising, insulin spike. In fact, beef and cheese cause a bigger insulin release than pasta, and fish produces a bigger insulin release than popcorn." Personally, I was thrilled to hear this, because I love nothing more than a bowl of whole grain pasta with veggie sausage, peppers, and onions!

Junk the Junk

Of course, just because a food is technically vegan doesn't mean it's good for you. If you want to lose weight, you have to stay away from junk food. You know what junk food is. I don't have to explain it to you. Anything that's really sweet or fatty or super-addictive is junk food. Period. Even if it's vegan.

If you find yourself obsessed with some kind of munchy that you know isn't good for you, simply stop bringing it into the house. Some foods just have a crazy power over us and we're better off not exposing ourselves to their temptations.

In much the same way, before you consider having "just one piece of chicken" or "only one slice of cheese," consider that these particular foods are quite literally addictive. In the case of dairy products, there are casomorphins to consider. These are compounds produced in your digestive tract after you eat cheese and other dairy products. That's right, the root of the word *morphine* is in there and for good reason—cheese is really habit forming. Not only because the creamy, fatty texture is so comforting, but also because when the milk protein breaks down during digestion, it's converted to something chemically similar to morphine and you just want more. In the same way an alcoholic can be set off by just one drink, someone who can't give up cheese might want to consider dairy their trigger for out-of-control eating.

According to a 2009 study at the University of Texas Southwestern Medical Center at Dallas, fat from certain foods actually makes its way into the brain, where the fat molecules signal the body to overcome appetite-suppressing hormones. And also consider that you literally overstimulate the pleasure center in your brain with fatty, sweet, or salty food and just as with drugs you need increasingly more of these rich substances to feel satisfied. And in much the same way as a drug addict might feel, you get strung out by the constant craving and remain hopelessly unsatisfied. Just watch how your behavior unfolds after you eat certain foods; if it is out of control, ditch those foods. A moment of good flavors is not worth the roller-coaster ride it's apt to put you on. It may be difficult for the first few days of withdrawal, but your taste buds will adjust if you give them half a chance.

Forget about Calorie Counting

Here's some of the best news of all. When you eat a plant-based diet, you don't need to obsess about calories or grams of protein; you need not weigh your food or eat according to your blood type. You need not worry about calculating carbs or food combining or making sure you have enough of certain amino acids. You need only move away from eating animals and their by-products in favor of a hearty, fiber-rich, and nutrient-dense plant-based diet. Such a diet will give you all that you need, and prevent you from getting the stuff that will drag you down. Fatty foods (e.g. meat and dairy) are calorie dense. A fat gram has 9 calories in it, as opposed to a carbohydrate, which has only 4 calories per gram. By avoiding fats, you avoid a lot of calories. Plant (vegan) foods are naturally low in fat.

There are better things to do with your time on earth than worry about calculating fat or protein grams. That will take care of itself when you steer clear of animal protein and all the trouble that goes with it. Think of the great sages and achievers throughout time: they certainly weren't scientists at mealtime—they ate to live, and they had greater goals and pursuits than how much they could titillate their taste buds or how well they could analyze nutrition labels.

How Long Does It Take to Lose Weight and How Much Will You Lose?

When you're in the process of losing weight, it's important to remember that the extra weight didn't just come about overnight, and in the same manner, it will take some time to lose it. Patience is important—hard, but important—because anything that happens super rapidly simply won't last. Fortunately for some people starting a vegan diet, less patience may be required than for other diets. Some people find that when they start a vegan weight-loss regime, excess weight begins to drop off quite literally overnight.

Experts agree that safe weight loss generally occurs at the rate of 1 to 2 pounds per week. However, depending on how you were eating before switching to a whole foods, plant-based diet, weight loss can be more dramatic on a vegan diet, especially as your body goes through the introductory period, usually lasting anywhere from two weeks to a month, of ridding itself of toxins and substances that have built up and clogged the body over the years from eating a diet heavy in animal products and/or processed foods. In some instances, people initially lose as much as 3 to 4 pounds per week before leveling off.

One of the first things you'll notice will of course be looser clothing. Within a few weeks, the weight loss will be visible both to you and to others. These noticeable results are great motivation, and the relatively rapid pace of loss will help you reinforce your commitment.

A 2005 study by Dr. Barnard and other researchers, which measured the effects of a low-fat vegan diet on body weight,

Thermic Effect

found that people lost significant amounts of weight with no calorie counting. On average, the low-fat vegan diet adopters lost 13 pounds in 14 weeks. This phenomenon can be partly explained by the thermic effects of eating plant-based foods. Vegan diets are higher in complex carbohydrates which cause the body to release some calories as body heat during digestion (the thermic effect) rather than store it as fat. In fact a vegan diet includes a rich variety of foods that have a thermic effect (see list below). We sometimes get a thermic effect with animal protein, but we are also stuck with all the animal fat that comes with it.

A whole foods, plant-based diet causes you to burn calories 16 percent faster after meals for about three hours. This revving up of your metabolism causes gradual and healthy weight loss. The thermic effect alone does not *cause* the weight loss. What it does is help decrease the number of calories that are automatically converted into fat—stopping some fat before it starts. It's a natural process that is aided significantly by choosing a plant-based diet and hampered by a diet high in animal fats.

In this same vein, when you eat a plant-based diet you dramatically boost (by an average of 60 percent) activity of the enzyme carnitine palmitoyltransferase, responsible for shoveling the fat we eat into the furnaces (mitochondria) in our cells to be burned for energy. This may help explain why those eating vegan are so much slimmer. Another reason for the easy weight loss that comes with a plant-based diet is that fiber naturally calms the appetite: it leaves the stomach slowly, making us feel full longer, so we end up eating fewer calories overall.

Thermic Effect is foods that release
Calories as body heat instead of
storing Ca storing Calories as Fat

A CAUTION ABOUT "THERMOGENIC" SUPPLEMENTS

There are hundreds of supplements available that tout their ability to promote thermogenesis; however, the nutrients and minerals in foods work synergistically. That is, you'll see much better, more lasting results consuming a whole food, with all its micronutrients, than from just taking a pill.

The main ingredient in many of these supplements is actually caffeine, which may help suppress appetite (though not as much as you might think—it takes a pretty high dose to have any real effect on appetite suppression), but along with that you may experience the bad side effects of caffeine—anxiety, nervousness, and irritability; and those moods can make it harder to make good decisions about what to eat.

The other commonly used ingredient is ephedra, which has an even worse track record than caffeine. Ephedra increases your heart rate and blood pressure. And it's not even that effective at regulating appetite over a long period of time. Ephedra's risks are extremely high (heart attack, stroke, and death), and the sale of supplements containing ephedra is still illegal in the United States, though many websites still promote it.

In fact a 2008 FDA investigation found that some weight-loss pills actually contained undeclared prescription drugs in them, such as fluoxetine (Prozac), phenytoin (an antiseizure medication), and phenolphthalein (a suspected cancer-causing laxative agent), that in some instances greatly exceeded the recommended maximum dosages. So in addition to pills being ultimately useless, they could also be dangerous. Sorry, but long-term weight loss is rarely accomplished by simply taking a pill.

All vegetables, beans, and whole grains are good sources of both fiber and complex carbohydrates, while there isn't an animal food on the planet that contains any fiber or complex carbohydrate at all. Zero. Zilch.

Thermic foods!

A vegan diet is a rich source of foods that have a thermic effect. Some good sources of highly thermogenic plant-based protein (and fiber!) include:

- Tofu, seitan, tempeh
- Nuts, seeds
- Beans, legumes

Many vegetables are also thermogenic, including chile peppers like cayenne. Some thermogenic fruits and vegetables are:

- Lettuce (iceberg is the least nutritious—go for dark green varieties)
- Spinach
- Mushrooms
- Celery
- Asparagus
- Cruciferous vegetables (kale, cabbage, broccoli, cauliflower)
- Apples
- Berries
- Peaches
- Apricots
- Pears

The effect of fat on cells.

These foods vary in their thermic effects, but all of them will help your body burn fat and lose weight.

And Dr. Barnard explains the metabolism issue this way: Your body burns glucose—a natural and necessary sugar that comes from starchy foods like whole grains, vegetables, and beans—for fuel to power just about everything from your muscles to your brain. Here's the problem: Fat from food forms little globules inside your cells which can obstruct the glucose from getting inside the cells to do the work it's meant to do. We can't burn the glucose if it can't get into our cells, which results in a more sluggish metabolism. The trick is that if we boot the fat out of our cells (by not eating fatty foods), our energy—and metabolism—becomes supercharged.

Stop Buying the Protein Myth

A common myth that persists and persists is that it's difficult to get enough protein from a vegan diet. Let's just put that myth to rest. The fact is, people on the standard American diet (SAD) eat nearly *twice* the recommended daily amount of protein—which can actually be unhealthy. According to the U.S. Food and Nutrition Board, recommended protein intake should be calculated according to your weight and age; it recommends 0.8 grams of protein per kilo of body weight, meaning that the average woman requires approximately 50 grams of protein per day, 56 grams for the average man. These guidelines also indicate that the preferred form of protein is from nonanimal sources, such as beans, legumes, nuts, and seeds. These protein sources are also naturally lower in fat, too, again supporting your weight loss efforts. Most of the fats they do contain are unsaturated and they're always cholesterol free.

To put it more simply, your average daily protein intake should be about 15 to 20 percent of your total daily calories (other sources say it can be even less—more like 10.7 percent)—a number easy to get to on a plant-based diet. There is protein in just about everything. So as long as you are eating a varied diet of whole grains, beans, and legumes, vegetables, fruits, and meat and dairy alternatives, you will be just fine.

No, there is absolutely no need to consume animal foods to get enough protein. In fact the American Dietetic Association holds that vegan diets provide more than enough protein, even without any special food combinations. Nutritionists used to think you needed to eat "complementary proteins"— beans *and* rice, for example—in one sitting to get all the nutrients we needed. We now know that's not true. As long as you are eating a bit of everything throughout the day, all is well.

Protein should account for about 15%–20% of your total daily calories—a number easy to get to on a plant-based diet.

When looking at the protein picture, it's important to consider what the Harvard School of Public Health calls the "protein package"—the saturated fats that come along with all meats, even so-called lean meat. You might find it surprising that skinless roasted chicken breast—the leanest chicken that could be, and way leaner than other meats—has 20 percent of its calories in fat, and 29 percent of which is saturated. That same 3-ounce piece of chicken also has 73 milligrams of cholesterol. According to the Harvard School of Public Health, only 7 percent *or less* of our daily fat intake should be from saturated fats. Eating animal protein makes consuming a low-fat, especially low-*saturated* fat, diet very difficult and a cholesterol-free diet impossible.

The best way to progress toward your ideal weight is to increase your intake of thermogenic foods without also increasing your intake of fats. Just follow this basic rule of thumb: If it's a whole grain, bean, fruit, or vegetable, you can eat as much of it as you want—and as long as you are not also piling on fat-rich animal foods, you will watch the pounds melt off and stay off.

But don't just take it from me. Listen to what the renowned nutritional scientist and vegetarian advocate Dr. Dean Ornish has to say.

Straight from the Source:
Dean Ornish, MD, on Losing Weight

No one has done more peer-reviewed research on the subject of weight loss and overall health than Dr. Ornish. He sparked a revolution in cardiology by proving that heart disease could be reversed with lifestyle (diet) changes, and his current research is showing that those very changes also affect gene expression: in other words, it seems we can turn on or turn off genes that affect cancer, heart disease, and longevity. He is the founder and the president of the nonprofit Preventive

Medicine Research Institute and is a clinical professor of medicine at the University of California, San Francisco. I interviewed Dr. Ornish on weight loss and diet.

KF: It's widely believed that people lose weight fastest on a high protein diet. But is it true?
DO: Initially, they may lose more weight because they are losing water weight. But by the end of a year, the weight usually returns. In general, slower weight loss by eating more healthfully is more sustainable. Slow but steady wins the race.

Most Americans also eat too many refined carbohydrates. When they go on a typical high-protein diet, they reduce their intake of all carbohydrates, which for most Americans means they primarily reduce their intake of refined carbohydrates. This [in itself] helps them to lose weight.

Whenever I debated Dr. [Robert] Atkins before he died, he was usually described as the "low carb" doctor and I was the "low fat" doctor. But that was never accurate. I have always advocated that an optimal diet is lower in total fat, very low in "bad fats" (saturated fat, hydrogenated fats, and trans-fatty acids), high in "good carbs" (fruits, vegetables, whole grains, legumes, and soy products), low in "bad carbs" (sugar, white flour, processed foods), and with enough of the "good fats" (omega-3 fatty acids) and high-quality proteins.

There are clear benefits to reducing the intake of refined carbohydrates, especially in people who are sensitive to them. The solution is not to go from refined carbohydrates like pasta to pork rinds and from sugar to sausage, but to substitute refined bad carbs with unrefined good carbs.

An optimal diet is:

- very low in "bad fats": saturated fat (butter and other animal fats), hydrogenated fats, and trans-fatty acids (the kind found in margarine, vegetable shortening, and anything with partially hydrogenated vegetable oils in its ingredients list)
- high in "good carbs": fruits, vegetables, whole grains, legumes, and soy products
- low in "bad carbs": sugar, white flour, processed foods
- "good fats" (omega-3 fatty acids, such as the ones found in flax seeds, walnuts, and canola oil) and high-quality proteins.

Good carbs are naturally high in fiber. The fiber fills you up before you eat too much. For example, it's hard to get too many calories from eating apples or whole grains, because apples are naturally low in calories and high in fiber, so you feel full before you consume too many calories.

Also, the fiber in good carbs causes your food to be digested and absorbed into your bloodstream more slowly. This helps to regulate your blood sugar into a normal range—neither too high nor too low.

When whole wheat flour is processed into white flour, or brown rice into white rice, the fiber and bran are removed. This turns a "good carb" into a "bad carb." Why? Because when the fiber and bran are removed, there is nothing to slow the digestion or signal that the body is full.

whole wheat flour processed to white flour
Brown Rice to whole Rice = fiber + bran removed

A NOTE FROM KF: THERE'S NOTHING FISHY ABOUT THESE OMEGA-3s

You will often hear people say that fish oil is the best source of omega-3 fatty acids. While it may be true that we are better able to assimilate the omega-3s in fish oil than from traditional vegan sources like flax oil, we now have a wonderful alternative. It turns out that fish obtain omega-3s by eating algae. With this in mind, several supplement makers are now extracting EPA and DHA (two key components of omega-3s) directly from the algae. You no longer have to participate in harming the environment through industrial fishing or inflicting suffering on fish and "bycatch" (birds, turtles, and dolphins caught and killed in fishing nets), or expose yourself to high levels of PCB and mercury contamination just to get your best sources of omega-3s. This brilliant solution supports becoming a veganist with ease.

KF: How should one eat in order to lose weight?

DO: Mindfully. It's not just *what* you eat, but also *how* you eat that matters. Have you ever eaten a bag of popcorn while watching an intense movie? All your attention is focused on the movie—so you may look down and see that the bag of popcorn is empty. You got all the calories but little of the pleasure. In contrast, if you really pay attention to your food, savoring it as you would a fine wine, you have greatly enhanced pleasure with fewer calories. And pleasure is sustainable.

KF: What should be avoided?

DO: As described above, avoid refined carbohydrates, too much fat (especially trans fats, which cause weight gain), and processed foods.

KF: **Should we count calories? Fat grams? Carbs?**

DO: In my experience, if you eat predominantly a whole foods, plant-based diet that is naturally high in fiber and low in fat and in refined carbohydrates, and if you eat it mindfully, you don't have to count anything to lose weight. You feel full before you consume too many calories.

KF: **What are some of the health risks of being overweight?**

DO: Being overweight significantly increases the risk of virtually every chronic disease. Some authorities have said that obesity is now overtaking smoking as the most preventable cause of premature death.

KF: **How do you break through cravings for unhealthy food—because they really do have a hold on most of us!**

DO: As you begin to eat more healthfully, your taste preferences change. You begin to prefer foods that are more healthful. And you connect the dots between what you eat and how you feel—because these mechanisms are so dynamic, most people find that they feel so much better, so quickly, it reframes the reason for changing from living longer to feeling better.

KF: **What is a reasonable rate of weight loss?**

DO: In most cases, no more than three pounds per week.

KF: **What if we want to lose weight faster? Is there a healthy way to do it?**

DO: Do more exercise and meditation and eat smaller amounts of healthy foods and less salt. Regular exercise not only burns calories, it also raises your basal metabolic rate, the number of calories you burn while at rest. Thus, exercise helps you lose weight even when you're not exercising. Do some strength training as well as aerobic exercise. Walking a mile burns even more calories than running a mile. Exercise in ways that you enjoy, then you're more likely to do it. If it's fun, it's sustainable.

I also want to make the point that you have a spectrum of choices; it's not all or nothing. In our research, we learned something very powerful: the more you change, the better you feel and the more you heal. What's sustainable are joy, pleasure, and freedom.

If you go *on* a diet, sooner or later you're likely to go *off* a diet—because a diet is what you can't have and what you must do. Even more than feeling healthy, most people want to feel free and in control.

What matters most is your overall way of living and eating. If you indulge yourself one day, then eat healthier the next. If you forget to exercise or meditate one day, do more the next. You get the idea. It's a very compassionate approach.

Some of the most toxic emotions are guilt, humiliation, and shame. If you go on a diet or a lifestyle program and feel like you have to follow it rigidly, then you're setting yourself up for feeling guilty, humiliated, and ashamed. The language of behavioral modification often has a moralistic quality to it that turns off a lot of people (like "cheating" on a diet).

It's a small step from thinking of foods as "good" or "bad" to seeing yourself as a "good person" or a "bad person" if you eat them, and this creates downward spirals in a vicious cy-

Its no small leap from thinking of foods as good vs. bad to thinking of yourself that way

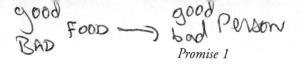
good food → good person
BAD bad

cle. For example, once you feel like you're a bad person for eating some ice cream, it's all too easy to say, "Well, I blew it, so I might as well finish the entire pint." Studies have shown that those who eat the healthiest overall are the ones who allow themselves some indulgences.

If you're trying to reverse heart disease or prevent the recurrence of cancer, you may need the "pound of cure"—that is, bigger changes in diet and lifestyle than someone who just wants to lower their cholesterol levels a few points or lose a few pounds. Offering a spectrum of choices is much more effective; then, you feel free. If you see your food and lifestyle choices each day as part of a spectrum, as a way of living, then you are more likely to feel empowered and to be successful.

KF: If someone is too busy to cook, and is in a big hurry, what is the best and most affordable approach?
DO: There are more and more healthy prepared and frozen meals on the market. Eat with your friends and take turns shopping and cooking—not only does it save time, but when you fill your heart with the love of friends and family in a shared meal, you have less need to overfill your belly.

For more information, you can visit Dr. Ornish's website at www.pmri.org.

Now let's meet someone who has put all this into play and transformed himself. Here's Ben Goldsmith's account of how he changed. I saw him recently at a party and didn't even recognize him. I'd seen pictures of him when he was heavier, and heard that he had a great weight-loss story, but the difference between then and now was astounding. Ben lost a total of 70 pounds, and he did it fairly effortlessly. His changes were motivated by health, but also by his ethics, a combination that seemed to work for him.

Ben Goldsmith's Story:
Weight Loss Was an Unexpected Benefit

Being overweight is difficult at any age, but it's particularly difficult, I think, for those of us who were overweight as children. Comments about our weight by strangers, family, and friends—however harmless they were intended to be—were incredibly painful reminders of a reality over which I had virtually no control and wanted so badly to change. As a kid I didn't know what *carbohydrate* or *calorie* meant. All I knew was I looked different from my friends, and I wanted more than anything to fit in.

I became self-conscious about my weight pretty early on. As a ten-year-old, I dreaded swimming lessons at summer camp because it meant taking off my shirt. I avoided looking down, particularly in pictures, because I knew it exaggerated my double chin. Riding on the school bus, I'd keep my knees together and try to take up as little space on the seat as possible.

My diet was never all that different from anyone else's. We mostly ate dinner at home and only had fast food occasionally. My parents packed the same ham and cheese sandwiches in my lunch that my friends' parents packed in theirs. But, for some reason, I always tended to be a little heavy.

Even though I had friends and a loving family, being overweight as a child made me feel sad and alone. It's a little hard to explain, but I always felt like I was different and that there was something wrong with me. The sadness went away when I did things that allowed me to forget about my body, and there were a few things that could always cheer me up. One of them was being around animals. Animals saw me the way I wanted to be seen: as a person just like anyone else.

Like many high schools around the country, my school allowed students to leave campus for lunch. And, like most schools in the United States, there were several fast-food restaurants within walking distance. Beginning in ninth grade, my friends and I ate fast food for lunch virtually every day. Not surprisingly, that's when I went from being heavier than my friends to being significantly overweight. By my junior year, at roughly five six, I weighed just over 200 pounds.

Having been overweight my entire life, I think at some point I just gave up. It didn't matter if I was a little heavy or seriously overweight. I was a fat kid and that wasn't going to change. The best I could do was eat the food my friends ate; at least that way I'd be one of them. At one point during my sophomore year, my friends invented a weekly event they called Meat Fest. Meat Fest, held at lunch on Fridays, entailed eating as much of as many different kinds of meat as we possibly could. My Meat Fest meal of choice: A double bacon cheeseburger with gyro meat and sausage from a local fast-food joint that was conveniently located on the same block as my high school. With fries and a Coke, I think it probably cost around $7.

I was never a particularly sedentary kid, mind you, even during the glory days of Meat Fest. All of this happened prior to the proliferation of wireless Internet connections, high school kids with cell phones, and Xbox Online. Hell, I was on the tennis team! I was a normal American kid eating normal American food doing normal American things. As I would come to find out a couple of years later, low and behold, the problem wasn't how often I ate or how little I exercised. The problem was the food I chose to eat.

On a spring day during my junior year of high school, my friend Katie and I had plans to catch a movie after school, and she'd invited a friend of hers, Ryan, to come along. The plan was to pick up Ryan on the way to the theater, and Katie and I decided to stop at McDonald's before heading to his house. While we were eating, Katie told me that Ryan ate a vegan diet, and she insisted we keep our stop at McDonald's a secret.

This struck me as odd. As far as I was concerned, we weren't doing anything wrong. I'd heard that

PETA was boycotting KFC at the time, and I would have understood the need for secrecy if we'd been eating there, but this was McDonald's—what could be so wrong about that? Still, the last thing I wanted to do was offend him, so I gladly agreed to keep our lunch between us.

Later we went back to Ryan's house and hung out. He seemed like a cool guy, and we had a lot in common. Nothing about Ryan suggested that his beliefs were fundamentally different from mine. Ryan offered Katie and me something to drink after a while: he had OJ, Coke, bottled water, and rice milk. I'd never heard of rice milk, so I asked if I could give it a try. It wasn't the best thing I'd ever tasted, but it wasn't bad either.

Why, I wondered, would this guy my own age deprive himself of a glass of milk, a Big Mac, or a plate of cheese fries? Given how much I enjoyed those things, his decision to abstain based on a set of beliefs actually struck me as rather commendable. He had to feel pretty strongly about it to refuse something so delicious. So I asked him why he chose to be vegan. His answer—that he wasn't willing to cause suffering to other living creatures, and then his recitation of lots of intense and awful details about that suffering—changed my life.

Effective that day, I was vegan, and have been ever since. It just made sense. Why should I eat something that caused an animal to suffer when I could choose to buy something else? Rice milk wasn't as good as milk, I thought, but it wasn't bad enough to justify buying cow's milk, which, as Ryan explained, came from an animal that was continually impregnated to maximize her dairy production, and her male calves were likely slaughtered for veal.

My decision to adopt a vegan diet was a very personal one. While I became increasingly concerned—and, later, outspoken—about the plight of animals raised on factory farms, I chose to adopt a vegan diet that day because I knew it was something I had the power to do, and I knew the choice was right for me. I loved Meat Fest as much as any of my friends, but I liked a lot of other foods, too. The way I saw it, when I sat down to eat, I could make a choice: I could eat the thing that I thought would taste best, or I could eat something perhaps slightly less delicious but that caused far less suffering. When I chose the latter, I felt good about myself—like in some small way I was making a difference.

I don't think I substantially changed what I ate on a daily basis; I replaced the animal products I'd been eating with plant-based alternatives. Rice or soy milk on cereal, PB&J instead of ham and cheese, Earth Balance instead of butter, tofu and seitan instead of meat. Except for the occasional temptation—a tiny slice of brie, my grandmother's matzo ball soup and coffee cake—I found that nearly everything I liked to eat could be replaced by a plant-based version of the same thing. Even when I tried a vegan product that tasted terrible, there was usually another brand that I found to be a little tastier. And, over time, vegan sour cream stopped tasting like, well, fake sour cream. Today, vegan sour cream tastes rich and creamy—a great topping for, or ingredient in, some of my favorite foods.

After a while, I stopped comparing the food I was eating as a vegan to the food I ate growing up. My tastes started to change. I had fewer cravings for rich and fatty foods, and I realized for the first time how sweet and satisfying whole foods can be. I started eating more fruits and nuts, used pure maple syrup as a sweetener instead of sugar, and added fresh spinach or kale to many of my favorite dishes. And, having never found a tofu scramble I really enjoyed, I invented my own.

My family was, by and large, supportive. My aunt Annie took me to a local bookstore to shop for vegan cookbooks and to read up on vegan nutrition. If my parents were cooking pasta with chicken for dinner, I'd just have my dad make me a serving without the chicken. If we were having tacos, I'd just have mine with beans, veggies, and salsa. Did I like beans as much as I liked ground beef and cheese? No. But it wasn't bad, I still got to eat with my family, and I felt good about my choices. And by the time I got to college, most grocery stores had begun stocking various plant-based meat and dairy replacements.

Even my friends were supportive. I still attended Meat Fest, and a double veggie burger and fries became my new usual. When we'd have barbecues over the summer, I'd bring along a box of Boca Burgers, and it was like nothing had changed at all. Sure, people cracked jokes about it, but they were my friends. I didn't object to what they ate and they didn't object to what I ate. We all just made our own choices, and no matter what anybody said, I felt good about mine.

Looking back on it now, it's amazing how little changed when I became vegan. It seems inconceivable that going from a meat eater one day to a vegan the next wouldn't require a huge shift in a person's life, but it certainly didn't in mine. There was one major thing that changed, but it was a change I didn't expect.

It never occurred to me that adopting a vegan diet would cause me to lose fifty pounds in two years, but that's what happened. I lost the first twenty or so pounds before I left for college. People were beginning to notice that I was slimming down, but I didn't notice a huge difference that first year until my mom took me shopping the summer before I left for my freshman year of college: I hadn't worn a size medium shirt or a pair of pants with a 34-inch waist since I started high school.

The rest of the weight came off my freshman year, and that's when the difference really became apparent. Gradually, over the course of that year, my body completely changed. My face looked slimmer, my waist leveled off at a size 32, and I even lost what my mother had always affectionately referred to as the "baby fat" on my hands.

Since the weight came off so slowly, it wasn't until I went home for Christmas that year that I fully understood the extent of the changes. My friends and family couldn't believe their eyes, and my grandmother found it rather unacceptable that I had yet to replace my new baggy clothes.

I didn't get substantially more exercise or eat any less than I ate before: I just ate differently. I'm virtually the same weight today as I was in my sophomore year of college, when for the first time in my life I finally felt good about my body, because I'd made changes in my diet that made me feel good about myself.

I love Ben's story because he got an unexpected benefit when he changed his diet to vegan. He made the switch because he loved animals, and the weight loss just came naturally, as a side effect. He demonstrates so well that "leaning in" to a new way of eating—in his case by "veganizing" his favorite foods—works easily.

I decided to lead with weight loss because it's an issue on so many people's minds, and they don't always know how easy it is to lose weight by cutting out animal-derived foods (and processed junk). That's the truth of it; when we choose to eat in ways that support our health and vitality, our bodies naturally find their ideal weight. (And if you don't need to lose weight, you won't; remember, your body has an inborn system of checks and balances that, once unburdened by the unnatural fatty diet full of animal protein, will keep you right where you are supposed to be.) The really great thing is that eating plant-based foods means you can ditch the scale and stop worrying about controlling every calorie and carb. On every level, your body will feel the difference. And, as you'll see when you turn to Promise 2, you'll be arming yourself against the great killer diseases of our time. Doesn't get much better than that!

PROMISE 2:

You Will Lower Your Risks for Cancer, Heart Disease, and Diabetes—and Even Reverse Diseases Already Diagnosed

Did you know?

- One out of every three children born after 2000 will develop type 2 diabetes, a disease preventable through diet and lifestyle choices.
- Animal protein (meat, dairy, and eggs) creates an acidic environment in the body, alters the mix of hormones to favor cell growth, modifies important enzyme activities to increase activation of carcinogens, and causes inflammation and cell proliferation—all of which create an ideal environment for cancer to thrive.
- You can reduce your chances of getting cancer by 40 percent, heart disease by 50 percent, and

diabetes by 60 percent by changing your diet to a whole foods, vegetarian diet.

- Within days of switching to a plant-based diet, weight starts to drop away; within a week, blood sugar starts to fall; within two weeks, blood pressure improves; and within a month, cholesterol improves significantly.
- Switching to a vegan diet and making some other important lifestyle changes (such as stress reduction and smoking cessation) seem to be *the* ticket to preventing and reversing major diseases.

You've heard it before: if things keep going the way they are, *half* of us will get cancer or heart disease and die from it. One out of every three children born after 2000 will develop type 2 diabetes, a disease that is almost entirely preventable. The diabetes epidemic is a rapidly emerging crisis, the seriousness of which I'm not sure we have yet recognized. The good news is, the means to prevent and heal disease seems to be right in front of us. It's in our food. Honestly, our food choices can either kill us—which mounting studies say that they are—or they can lift us right out of the disease process and into soaring health.

Here's what the latest science tells us: according to the Physicians Committee for Responsible Medicine, you can reduce your chances of getting cancer by 40 percent, heart disease by 50 percent, and diabetes by 60 percent simply by following a whole foods, vegetarian diet (the odds are even better when you cut out eggs and dairy), and these are conservative numbers. On top of this, a plant-based diet can help people with all these conditions recover more quickly and fully. And even more startling: such diets can be catalysts in *curing* some of the most serious diseases we face. That's right, *curing*.

Our food choices can either kill us—which mounting studies say that they are—or they can lift us right out of the disease process and into soaring health.

What this science is telling us is that we have to rethink all our assumptions about deadly diseases. No longer are pharmaceuticals or drastic medical procedures your only option; there is so much hope on your plate and in your pantry.

Shifting to a vegan diet and making some other important lifestyle changes (such as stress reduction and smoking cessation) seems to be *the* ticket to preventing, reversing, even curing disease.

Eating foods that support healing while cutting out foods that create havoc can change the course of your life.

In this chapter we'll look at cancer, heart disease, and diabetes in turn to better understand how what we eat can make a difference.

Conquering Cancer

I am very fortunate to know T. Colin Campbell, PhD, professor emeritus of Cornell University and coauthor of the ground-breaking *The China Study*. I strongly recommend this book; it's an expansive and hugely informative work on the effects of food on health. Campbell's work is regarded by many as the definitive epidemiological examination of the relationship between diet and disease. He has received more than seventy grant years of peer-reviewed research funding (the gold standard of research), much of it from the National Institutes of Health (NIH), and he has authored more than 300 research papers. Dr. Campbell grew up on a dairy farm and believed wholeheartedly in the health value of eating animal protein. Indeed, he set out in his career to investigate how to produce more and better animal protein. Troublesome to his preconceived opinion about the goodness of dairy, Campbell kept running up against results that pointed to a different truth: that animal protein is disastrous to human health.

Through a variety of experimental study designs, epidemiological evidence (studies of what affects the illness and health of populations), and observation of real-life conditions that had rational, biological explanations, Dr. Campbell has made a direct and powerful correlation between cancer and animal protein. For this book I asked Dr. Campbell to explain a little about how and why nutrition (both good and bad) affects cancer in our bodies.

He explains that at various times throughout our lives, cancer cells pop up in all of us. (Yes, you read that right.) But what "feeds" the cancer and fortifies it is, among other things, animal protein. Why is that? Because animal protein (all meat, dairy, and eggs) creates an acidic environment in the body, alters the mix of hormones to favor cell growth, modifies important enzyme activities to increase activation of carcinogens, and causes inflammation and cell proliferation—all of which creates an ideal environment for cancer to thrive.

On the other hand, when you eat a plant-based (vegan) diet, you are getting the antioxidants inherent in vegetables and fruits that are critical to neutralizing cancer-causing free radicals in the body, along with fiber, which acts like a scrub brush as it moves through your body. A varied, plant-based diet, he claims, is a protective diet—sufficient in amino acids for protein needs; high in fiber, antioxidants, vitamins, and minerals; and low in saturated fats.

The following is a conversation I had with Dr. Campbell to better understand this dynamic.

Straight from the Source:
T. Colin Campbell, PhD, on Diet and Cancer

KF: What happens in the body when cancer develops? What is the actual process?
TCC: Cancer generally develops over a long period of time, which can be divided into three stages: initiation, promotion, and progression.

Initiation occurs when chemicals or other agents attack the genes of normal cells to produce genetically modified cells capable of eventually causing cancer. The body generally repairs most such damage, but if the cell reproduces itself before it is repaired, its new (daughter) cell retains this genetic damage. This process may occur within minutes and, to some extent, is thought to be occurring most of the time in most of our tissues.

Promotion occurs when the initiated cells continue to replicate themselves and grow into cell masses that eventually will be diagnosed. This is a long growth phase occurring over months or years and is known to be reversible.

Progression occurs when the growing cancer masses invade neighboring tissues and/or break away from the tissue of origin (metastasis) and travel to distant tissues when they are capable of growing independently, at which point they are considered to be malignant.

KF: Why do some people get cancer and others don't? What percentage is genetic, and what percentage has to do with diet?
TCC: Although the initiated cells are not considered to be reversible, the cells growing through the promotion stage usually are, which is a very exciting concept. This is the stage that especially responds to nutritional factors. For example, the nutrients from animal-based foods, especially the protein, promote the development of the cancer, whereas the nutrients from plant-based foods, especially the antioxidants, reverse the promotion stage. This is a very promising observation because cancer proceeds forward or backward as a function of the balance of promoting and anti-promoting factors found in the diet. Thus, consuming anti-cancer-promoting, plant-based foods tends to keep the cancer from going forward, perhaps even reversing the promotion. The difference between individuals is almost entirely related to their diet and lifestyle practices.

Although all cancers and other diseases begin with genes, this is not the reason why the disease actually appears. If people do the right thing during the promotion stage, perhaps even during the progression stage, cancer will not appear, and if it does, it might even be resolved. Most estimates suggest that not more than 2 to 3 percent of cancers are due entirely to genes; almost all the rest is due to diet and lifestyle factors. [Note from Kathy: Which is not to say that anyone is to blame for "creating their cancer," but rather that we have a powerful tool available to us to prevent further damage and possibly to reverse the damage already in motion.]

The nutrients from animal-based foods, especially the protein, promote the development of the cancer, whereas the nutrients from plant-based foods, especially the antioxidants, reverse the promotion stage.
—T. Colin Campbell

Consuming plant-based foods offers the best hope of avoiding cancer, perhaps even reversing cancer once it is diagnosed. Believing that cancer is attributed to genes is a fatalistic idea, but believing that cancer can be controlled by nutrition is a far more hopeful one.

KF: You said that initially something attacks the genes— chemicals or other agents. Like what?
TCC: Cancer, like every other biological event—good or bad—begins with genes. In the case of cancer, gene[s] that

give rise to cancer either may be present when we are born or, during our lifetimes, normal genes may be converted into cancer genes by certain highly reactive chemicals (i.e., carcinogens).

Consider "cancer genes" as seeds that grow into tumor masses only if they are "fed." The "feeding" comes from wrongful nutrition. It's like growing a lawn. We plant seeds, but they don't grow into grass (or weeds) unless they are provided water, sunlight, and nutrients. So it is with cancer. In reality, we are planting seeds all throughout our lifetime, not only for cancer but also for other events as well. But this mostly does not matter unless we "nourish" their growth.

The chemicals that create these cancer genes are called carcinogens. Most carcinogens of years past have been those that attack normal genes to create cancer genes. These are initiating carcinogens, or initiators. But more recently, carcinogens also may be those that promote cancer growth. They are promoting carcinogens, or promoters.

Our work showed that casein, an animal protein widely used in research studies, is the most relevant cancer promoter ever used in a laboratory. This striking research observation was then used to investigate whether it was consistent with practical diets, and we found, both biochemically and epidemiologically, that all diets rich in animal foods and low in whole plant-based foods had the same effect, thus indicating all animal protein, not just casein.

The most important point to consider is that we cannot do much about preventing initiation, but we can do a lot about preventing promotion.

KF: What exactly is so bad about animal protein?
TCC: I wouldn't say "exactly," because it suggests something very specific. Rather, animal protein causes a broad spectrum of adverse effects.

Among other fundamental effects, it makes the body more acidic, alters the mix of hormones, and modifies important enzyme activities, each of which can cause a broad array of more specific effects. One of these effects is its ability to promote cancer growth (by operating on key enzyme systems, by increasing hormone growth factors, and by modifying the tissue acidity). Another is its ability to increase blood cholesterol (by modifying enzyme activities) and to enhance atherogenesis, which is the early stage of cardiovascular disease.

KF: Okay, so I am clear that it's wise to avoid casein, which is intrinsic in dairy (milk and cheese), but how is other animal protein, such as chicken, steak, or pork, implicated in the cause and growth of cancer?

Casein, which is a protein in dairy products, is the most relevant cancer promoter ever discovered.

TCC: I would first say that casein is not just "intrinsic" but *is the main protein of cow milk, representing about 87 percent of the milk protein.*

The biochemical systems that underlie the adverse effects of casein are also common to other animal-based proteins.

Also, the amino acid composition of casein, which is the characteristic primarily responsible for its cancer-promoting property, is similar to most other animal-based proteins. They all have what we call high "biological value," in comparison, for example, with plant-based proteins, which is why animal protein promotes cancer growth and plant protein doesn't.

KF: Isn't anything in moderation okay, as long as we don't overdo it?
TCC: I rather like the expression used by my friend Caldwell Esselstyn, the Cleveland Clinic surgeon who reversed heart disease and who says, "Moderation kills!" I prefer to go the whole way, not because we have foolproof evidence showing that 100 percent is better than, say, 95 percent for every single person for every single condition, but that it is easier to avoid straying off on an excursion that too often becomes a slippery slope back to our old ways. Moreover, going the whole way allows us to adapt to new unrealized tastes and to rid ourselves of some old addictions. And finally, moderation often means very different things for different people.

KF: Are you saying that if one changes their diet from animal-based protein to plant-based food that the disease process of cancer can be halted and reversed?
TCC: Yes, this is what our experimental research shows. I also have become aware of many anecdotal claims by people who have said that their switch to a plant-based diet stopped or even reversed their disease. One study on melanoma has been published in the peer-reviewed literature that shows convincing evidence that it is substantially halted with this diet.

Switching to a plant-based diet, even after years of poor nutrition, may halt cancer growth.

KF: How long does it take to see changes?
TCC: It is not clear, because carefully designed research in humans has not been done. However, we demonstrated and published findings showing that experimental progression of disease is at least suspended, and even reversed, when tumors are clearly present.

KF: Consider a person who has been eating poorly his whole life; is there still hope that a dietary change can make a big difference? Or is everything already in motion?
TCC: A variety of evidence shows that cancers and noncancers alike can be stopped even after a person has consumed a poor diet earlier in life. This effect is equivalent to treatment, a very exciting concept.

KF: This is sounding like it's something akin to a cure; is that the case?
TCC: Yes. The problem in this area of medicine is that traditional doctors are so focused on the use of targeted therapies (chemo, surgery, radiation) that they refuse to even acknowledge the use of therapies like nutrition and are loath to even do proper research in this area. So, in spite of the considerable evidence—theoretical and practical—to support a

beneficial nutritional effect, every effort will be made to discredit it. It's a self-serving motive.

KF: What else do you recommend we do to avoid, stop, or reverse cancer?
TCC: A good diet, when coupled with other health-promoting activities like exercise, adequate fresh air and sunlight, good water, and sleep, will be more beneficial. The whole is greater than the sum of its parts.

   *Just a note here: This is very exciting information, but it is in no way encouragement to refuse traditional treatment. If you are dealing with cancer, please make your health and medical decisions with your doctor.

   What sticks with me more than anything is the concept that animal protein could feed cancer cells like fertilizer feeds a lawn. So those chicken patties and barbecue ribs I grew up loving literally help cancer grow in the body. This is a subject that means a lot to me because I have so much cancer in my family—my father died from melanoma at sixty-four—and I often wonder how a good healthy diet might have changed the course of things for him. I feel so empowered knowing that there is such a practical, effective thing we can do to fight cancer: we can change our diet from an animal-based one to a plant-based one. We can eat all those colorful fruits and vegetables and reap the rewards of the vitamins and antioxidants therein. Very exciting!

   In addition to what Dr. Campbell has shared, many studies show that women who are overweight are at greater risk for succumbing to breast cancer. Trimming away extra weight helps them survive. And as discussed earlier, plant-based diets make weight control much easier.

But the promise of a healthy diet goes even further. The Women's Intervention Nutrition Study, which included 2,437 postmenopausal women who had previously been treated for breast cancer, tested whether a low-fat diet could reduce the risk that cancer might recur. And it did. In this study, most of the participants simply cut down on meat and other fatty foods, and it remains to be seen whether going further—eliminating these products completely—would be even more effective.

Adding physical exercise helps too. In the Women's Healthy Eating and Living Study, which included approximately 3,000 women, all of whom had been treated for breast cancer, those who had at least five daily servings of fruits and vegetables and averaged thirty minutes of walking each day had roughly half the mortality risk, compared with women who ate fewer vegetables and fruits or who were less active.

Diet also makes a huge difference for men. Dr. Dean Ornish, who had already shown the ability of a low-fat vegetarian diet, along with other lifestyle measures, to reverse heart disease, tested a similar diet for men with prostate cancer. To track their progress, he used a blood test for prostate-specific antigen (a rapidly rising PSA is a sign of advancing cancer). Dr. Ornish showed that, on average, men who avoided animal products actually had a drop in their PSA levels, meaning their cancer was not advancing and might actually be retreating. Meanwhile, the cancers of men in a control group who made no diet changes continued to worsen.

Putting these studies together, the healthiest combination

appears to be to cut out fatty foods—especially animal products—boost vegetables and fruits, and lace up your sneakers.

The scientific community is still trying to verify the straight line between a vegan diet and cancer *cures* (once someone has cancer, there are a million variables that can't be easily accounted for, and diet is difficult both to isolate and to enforce). That said, there is a growing body of anecdotal evidence of people staving off cancer by turning to a plant-based diet (along with other healthy practices, of course).

Next you'll meet Meg Wolff, whose cancer has been halted, largely, she believes, because she eliminated animal foods from her diet and chooses whole, fresh, plant-based foods instead.

Meg Wolff's Story:
Surviving Cancer with a Plant-Based Diet

I think it's fair to say that for about the first half of my life, I didn't think much about the effects of any foods I put into my body. Most people don't. Growing up in Westbrook, Maine, in the 1960s, I of course ate whatever my mother served—meat as the main course, frozen or fresh veggies, home-baked desserts, lots of milk. This was what was considered healthy at that time.

As a teen, I ditched the vegetables and got addicted to fast-food cheeseburgers, fries, and milkshakes. I'd often use my lunch money for a bag of salty chips, a candy bar, a pastry, and a diet soda! Like kids today, once I got a taste for processed sweets and foods, nothing healthy satisfied me.

Over the next few years, I had intense menstrual cramps, a racing heartbeat that required medication, psoriasis for which I took cortisone and tar baths, and bouts of diarrhea. I bounced back easily from each of these things, though, and lived a very active, otherwise healthy life. I always considered myself the strong, fit one in my family. So I never paused to consider what might have caused these illnesses.

I was introduced to the concept of food as medicine in 1982, when my husband Tom and I lived in Korea right after getting married. My Korean friends tried to impress upon me the need to take care of and protect my body with appropriate foods, but I was too blinded by my Western upbringing to embrace this message. After three years in Korea, we moved to Portland, Oregon. By that point I had been living with pain in the back of my knee for several years, but doctors always wrote it off as nothing to worry about and prescribed pain relievers. Over the next couple of years, the pain really started to bother and limit me. At age thirty-three, I was diagnosed with bone cancer that required me to have my left leg amputated above the knee.

We had just bought our first home in a great neighborhood. I was happily staying home to raise my kids. I had a four-year-old son whom I loved taking to the playground, and my new baby daughter woke up every morning with a big smile on her face. And then . . . BAM! The cancer came and my vibrantly colored world turned into one the color of a brown paper bag. Gone was the feeling that I wanted to ride with the car windows open and sing with the radio. "Devastated" doesn't begin to cover what I felt.

After I lost my leg, I was drawn to the subject of food and health. I read books about how diet could be used to help eliminate cancer from the body, and I consulted a naturopathic doctor. The naturopath recommended dietary changes, including eliminating dairy. But still, the power of food was largely lost on me. I did add more whole grains and vegetables to our diet and cut back on sugar, but I continued eating meat, cheese, and ice cream. Soon after, I had more bowel problems. I figured my system couldn't handle the extra grains and veggies, so I stopped eating them.

Once I had a reasonably comfortable prosthetic leg, I was ready to catch up on life, and my whole family got involved with skiing. It turned out we were all pretty good at it, including me! Still, though, sinus issues and headaches that I'd always chalked up to the damp Oregon weather remained. A specialist prescribed antibiotics—and that led to debilitating ulcerative colitis. To top it off, at various doctor appointments I'd ask about lumps I was feeling under my arms and in my breasts. Doctors called it fibrocystic breast disease, acted unconcerned, and advised annual mammograms.

By 1998, the lumps had become more numerous, and I again brought this to my doctor's attention. Again, I was told not to worry.

Between the prescription drugs and my leg, I was often exhausted and depressed. And I had a growing fear about my breasts. I tried to let it go—until I discovered a protruding hard lump in my right breast. My doctor shrugged it off, attributing it to my crutches likely shifting a swollen lymph node. I sought a referral and, after testing, the specialist too told me not to worry.

We were just getting ready to move back to Maine, where my mother was very sick with colon cancer. I had so many other things to take care of. Besides, I told myself, lightning couldn't strike twice, right? I mean, what were the chances that I'd have another cancer?

These thoughts kept me from freaking out, but as it turned out, the chances were really remarkable: We moved to Maine in June, my mother died in July, and in December, at age forty-one, I was diagnosed with stage 3B invasive breast cancer.

I had surgery in January 1999 to remove my right breast. It was painful, physically and especially emotionally. Tom and I already had weathered so much, and I worried about our ability to get through another huge thing and be happy again. I started my chemotherapy treatments with a heavy heart, knowing my doctors weren't hopeful about a long-term remission. I worried about dying and leaving my children.

And then, between chemo sessions, I finally found some real hope. I visited another naturopath, and this time I was finally ready to heed her advice. She said that eating a plant-based diet had helped some women with breast cancer. All of a sudden, a light went on. I finally connected the dots.

Between treatments, I mustered up the energy to buy some whole grains and vegetables. I couldn't learn enough fast enough! I happily cooked my healthy food, and it felt right. I signed up for cooking classes. I dove in. At first, many family members and friends thought I had really lost my mind because I believed this food was going to help heal my close-to-death body.

As I was about to start radiation treatments, the radiologist took one look at me and advised me to prepare my soul to die. But I had other plans.

I continued cooking and eating my plant-based foods, and I quickly started to feel much better. I had more energy. I didn't need sleeping pills to sleep through the night. I was less anxious. Despite having regular radiation treatments, I felt better than I had in years—like the world was finally right-side up. After a year and a half of eating well, I was off all medications for the first time in more than a decade. My chemo and radiation treatments were over, and my health was excellent. My doctors and I were in awe. When I first switched to a plant-based diet, it just made sense in my soul, so I took a leap of faith. I grew to love the food and the healthy lifestyle I was leading. I then educated myself about the science that backs up a plant-based diet by taking classes and voraciously reading.

As I started improving and stayed healthy, my doctors liked to say I was a miracle patient. But I knew I had, at least in part, made my own luck. It's been twelve years, and I've never looked back. I consider it my life's work now to share this message—that what we eat matters most, that you can maintain or regain your good health by eating a plant-based diet!

You can get some of Meg Wolff's healing recipes in her book *A Life In Balance: Healthy Recipes from Maine.* I am grateful to Meg for sharing her story. I hear stories like hers often, and they offer such hope. Just think about what is yet to be discovered about the link between foods and cancer. I strongly suspect we will soon have conclusive, irrefutable evidence that we've been eating ourselves to death with our high-fat, animal-based diets. But let me be clear. In no way am I suggesting that changing your diet is the only thing that will and does make a difference with cancer. As always, if you have cancer or feel a lump somewhere or notice an odd-looking mole, talk with your doctor about all your treatment options, do your own reading, and set about your journey with a well-rounded approach.

Halting Heart Disease

When you have heart disease, or are approaching it, it's like there is a war going on in your body. You likely have high blood pressure, which assaults your heart, rapidly wearing it out. Quite often, heart disease goes right along with obesity, and that means you have miles of extra blood vessels going out to nourish your extra-large body, and your heart struggles to keep up.

The exciting news is that within days of making a diet change, weight starts to drop away. Within a week, blood sugar starts to fall. Within two weeks, blood pressure improves. Within a month, cholesterol improves significantly.

You see a reduced need for medications, and less risk of the complications associated with them.

Perhaps the most widely recognized advantage of cutting out meat and dairy is what it does for your heart. Dr. Dean Ornish revolutionized cardiology when his studies indicated that the blocked arteries of 82 percent of his participating patients could be opened if they switched to a vegetarian diet (along with other lifestyle changes such as meditation and support groups).

Switch to a plant-based, vegan diet and within days weight starts to drop away, within a week blood sugar starts to fall, within two weeks blood pressure improves, and within a month cholesterol improves significantly. Research shows that a vegetarian diet could add a good ten years onto your life.

Dr. Caldwell Esselstyn, a researcher and clinician at the Cleveland Clinic for over thirty-five years, says emphatically, "If the truth be known, coronary artery disease is a toothless paper tiger that need never, ever exist, and if it does exist it need never, ever progress." In 1991, Dr. Esselstyn served as the president of the American Association of Endocrine Surgeons and organized the first National Conference on the Elimination and Prevention of Heart Disease. In 2005, he became the first recipient of the Benjamin Spock Award for Compassion in Medicine. Dr. Esselstyn is also an Olympic gold medalist in rowing, and he was awarded the

Bronze Star as an army surgeon in Vietnam. Here is what I learned from him.

Straight from the Source:
Caldwell Esselstyn, MD, on Heart Disease

KF: What exactly is coronary heart disease?
CE: Coronary heart disease is the leading killer of women and men in Western civilization. It is predicted to become the number one global disease burden by 2020.

It consists of an inflammatory buildup of blockages in arteries to the heart muscle. These blockages are made of fat, cholesterol, calcium, and inflammatory cells. Blockages can become severe enough to cause symptoms such as shortness of breath or chest pain (angina). When blockages suddenly become complete, the portion of heart muscle fed by that blocked artery is now deprived of oxygen and nutrients, thus it is injured or dies. This is a heart attack. The patient may survive or succumb if the event is accompanied by a fatal heart rhythm.

KF: Who develops heart disease?
CE: Just about anyone eating the typical Western diet. In autopsy studies of our GIs who died in the Vietnam and Korean wars, almost 80 percent, at an average age of just twenty years old had disease that could be seen without a microscope. Forty years later, in 1999, a study of young persons between the ages of sixteen and thirty-four who had died in accidents, homicides, and suicides found that disease is now ubiquitous.

KF: What is the cause of the disease?
CE: It is the typical Western diet of processed oils, dairy, and meat, which destroys the life jacket of our blood vessels—our endothelial cells. This cell layer is the one-cell-thick lining of all our blood vessels. Endothelial cells manufacture a magical protective molecule of gas called nitric oxide, which protects our blood vessels. It keeps our blood flowing smoothly, it is the strongest dilator (widener) of our blood vessels, it inhibits the formation of blockages (plaques), and it inhibits inflammation.

KF: With such natural protection, why do we ever develop heart disease?
CE: Every Western meal of processed vegetable oils, dairy products, and meat (including chicken and fish) injures these endothelial cells. As individuals consume these damaging products throughout their lives, they have fewer functioning endothelial cells remaining and thus less of the protective nitric oxide. Without enough nitric oxide the plaque blockages build up and grow, eventually creating heart disease and strokes.

KF: Can it be stopped or even reversed?
CE: Yes. First we must look at the lessons learned from cultures such as those in rural China, the Highlands of Papua New Guinea, central Africa, and the Tarahumara people of northern Mexico, where there is a virtual absence of coronary artery heart disease. Their nutrition is plant based and without oil.

Beginning in 1985 I initiated a study of seriously ill coronary artery disease patients. I put them on a plant-based diet, without any oil. Their cholesterol levels plummeted. Their angina disappeared. Their weight dropped. I have reported this study at five years, twelve years, and sixteen years, in the peer-reviewed scientific literature and again beyond twenty years in my book *Prevent and Reverse Heart Disease*. In some of the patients we had follow-up angiograms (Xrays) of previously blocked arteries demonstrating striking disease reversal.

The greatest gift to these patients is the increasing recognition that they are the locus of control for their disease—not some pill or procedure. They have made themselves heart-attack-proof and lose the greatest fear of all heart patients and their families—when will the next one occur?

KF: What about drugs, stents, and heart bypass surgery?
CE: In the midst of a heart attack a stent or bypass may be lifesaving, however, for the remaining 90 percent of patients, studies confirm that they do not prevent future heart attacks or prolong life. They are associated with significant complications such as hemorrhage, heart attack, stroke, cognitive decline, depression, and death. The benefits erode with the passage of time as the stents and bypasses may themselves develop blockage.

"Stents may be lifesaving *during* a heart attack, but they do not prevent future heart attacks or prolong life."
—Dr. Caldwell Esselstyn

Some drugs may decrease blood pressure and the heart workload. Others interfere with clotting, which helps a stent remain open. Statin drugs lower cholesterol. None of these drugs or interventions addresses the basic causation of disease, and not surprisingly, the disease progresses with the need for more drugs, stents, and repeat bypasses.

KF: Why aren't physicians using nutrition therapy?
CE: Most physicians have no training or understanding of the power of nutrition. In a busy practice they would not have the time for it. It is my belief that physicians must accord the plant-based lifestyle transition its due. Every patient with cardiovascular disease should be referred to a physician or nurse practitioner with the knowledge and expertise in these counseling skills.

KF: Any final thoughts?
CE: When people learn to eat plant-based, to eliminate heart disease, it could inaugurate a seismic revolution in their overall health. Other diseases that resolve include obesity, hypertension, stroke, gallstones, diverticulitis, asthma, osteoporosis, allergies, rheumatoid arthritis, multiple sclerosis, lupus, and studies have shown a marked decrease in the common Western cancers of breast, prostate, colon, endometrial, ovarian, and pancreatic.

"Plant-based eating could inaugurate a seismic revolution in health."—Dr. Caldwell Esselstyn

---

Now you know how heart disease happens from a medical viewpoint. Here is one man's personal story. Actually, it's three stories woven into one.

Robert Dew's Story:
Reversing the Family Heart-Attack Pattern

For the record, this is a portion of my family's health history:

> Great-uncle: deceased at 45. Cause: heart attack.
> Grandfather: deceased. Cause: heart attack.
> Grandmother: deceased. Cause: stroke.
> Great-grandfather: deceased. Cause: heart attack.
> Mother: deceased. Cause: congestive heart failure.
> Father: living with two triple bypasses, two pacemakers, and congestive heart failure.

That's how my family stories end. We all die of heart attacks and strokes. But every story has a beginning, too . . .

I recall a set of stemware from my childhood—a nice set of sturdy, faceted goblets. They were obtained courtesy of a well-known peanut butter manufacturer. The peanut butter came off the shelf in special glasses, sealed with a pry-off lid. Our set was a result of my eating countless spoons of it in front of the TV. We had an even dozen. I would have been pleased to supply a dozen more, but the promotion ended.

I had another food treat, this one invented by my dad. He would sit down to watch a football game with a stick of butter, a packet of saltines, and a bottle of ginger ale. He scraped out a furrow of butter onto the cracker and downed the thing in one bite. Every two or three of these were washed down with ginger ale. I loved it too. By halftime, the butter, crackers, half a jar of peanut butter, and a quart of ginger ale were gone. We were eagerly consuming the three main food groups in the American Food Pyramid: sugar, grease, and salt.

I did eat other things. I loved breakfast; listening to bacon and eggs talk to me as they cooked in the same pan. Grits had to be consumed with a ton of butter, salt, and pepper. Hamburgers were my favorite food. I always took off the lettuce and tomato and gave the pickle to my wife. I could not pass a hamburger stand without wanting to stop for double fries and triple burgers. When I cooked burgers on the grill (which was often) I always made an extra rare and greasy one to eat while I was cooking the rest. I did like broccoli, as long as it was rendered unrecognizable, swimming in butter and cheese. Then there were doughnuts; fried in oil, dripping hot from the basket, coated in sugar. And more than once, at midnight, I found myself eating Oreo cookies while staring at the clock. So there you have it: breakfast, lunch, supper, dessert, and snacks—a diet of kings.

I ate a lot of fast food, and dined at other restaurants. When we ate at home there was plenty of meat and potatoes. Of course we added a tiny feel-good garnish of fruits and vegetables that were either loaded with sugar or cooked in some sort of fat. I went to the gym and took vitamins. But while I was eating all this, I was doing something else; I was constructing, piece by piece, the links of a chain. The resulting concatenation: heart disease.

Awakening

My awakening was gradual. I had been watching my father take a seemingly inexorable journey. During each of his bypass surgeries I witnessed drops in his cognitive skills. This once sharp and inventive man was moving backward. Holding the thread of a simple conversation became difficult. In parallel with this was an increasingly diminished physical capacity. The strong man of my youth was growing feeble. In many ways our roles were reversing; the child became parent and caregiver. But it made me think . . .

A few years ago I started to consider my position. In thinking about my dad, I remembered reading an article in the late '70s about a treatment that reversed heart disease through diet—the Nathan Pritikin diet. While researching his methods I found other books that detailed the relationship between the typical Western diet and degenerative diseases—books by Ross Horne, Dean Ornish, Caldwell Esselstyn, and Lance Gould. I tried to practice the lifestyle, but could not maintain it.

Then it happened to me. I became aware of symptoms consistent with heart disease. Once they began, they progressed at an alarming rate. I contacted Dr. Esselstyn and described my symptoms. I had already read his book and asked if he could recommend a doctor who supported his method of treatment. In July 2009, I went to a clinic and had a stress echo test. I failed miserably.

The attending nurses and doctor wanted to send me to the hospital immediately to have a catheterization and most likely a stent or bypass. I told the attending doctor that I respected his opinion but that I had to put on the brakes. I had already concluded that I wanted to try a plant-based solution to my problem. Needless to say, that announcement caused some hysteria.

Treatment

Dr. Esselstyn supported the decision. I was immediately armed with nitroglycerin tablets and instructed to go to the hospital if I had to use them. Beta blockers and statin medications became part of my daily regimen and I renewed my dedication to a plant-based diet. As it turned out, there was a cancellation and subsequent opening in what was Dr. Esselstyn's first small-group program at the Cleveland Clinic's newly opened wellness center.

This was my condition just prior to stress echo testing:

- Blood pressure: resting, 130/95.
- Cholesterol: 250.
- I had to stop three times on my way to the test from the hospital parking lot. No hills or steps; I was on level ground.

- During walks with my grandchildren, I could make two driveways before angina onset.
- I could no longer maintain my former fast walking pace.
- I couldn't wrestle on the living room floor with the grandkids.
- I had excessive weight gain. Waist size 38 inches, pushing 200 pounds at 5'7".
- Emotional and work stress could trigger angina attacks.
- I had to take an acid reducer every day or suffer severe indigestion.
- My joints ached; I was stiff every morning.
- I'd had acne rosacea since puberty, and my skin was worsening every year. (I like to joke that I had four of the new seven dwarves: Flaky, Oily, Blotchy, and Red.)
- I had developed tinnitus (ringing in the ears) during the previous year. It was worsening.

I attended Dr. Esselstyn's program in early August 2009. Since then, I have had no surgical intervention. The approach has been through diet and regular moderate cardio exercise. The diet is totally plant-based with no added fats or oils. Beginning gradually, after about a week into my new lifestyle, and over the course of six months, my physical conditions changed to:

- Blood Pressure: resting, 115/65.
- Cholesterol: 127.

- I was no longer stopping halfway through parking lots.
- I walked around the block with my grandkids without discomfort, and I wasn't counting driveways.
- I walked at my old fast pace again.
- I could wrestle with the grandkids again.
- Emotional and work stress did not trigger angina.
- I lost about 35 pounds, back into a 32-inch waist.
- I stopped taking acid reducers. No indigestion.
- My morning stiffness and joint aches almost completely stopped.
- My acne has cleared up beyond what I could ever have imagined.
- I've experienced a perceptible reduction in the volume of the tinnitus.

As far as I am concerned, the results are nothing short of miraculous. That's my story, but my story is really three stories.

Collateral Benefits

My wife Barbara had a heart attack two and a half years ago, had a stent implanted, and went through subsequent cardiac rehabilitation. She was faithful about exercise and stayed close to the doctors' recommended diet (although, I myself found it perplexing that hamburgers were on the menu in the recovery room). All the previous symptoms had gone; she had no edema in her feet, no shortness of breath, no chest pain.

About four or five months after surgery she had an angina attack. That was only the first. The angina episodes returned with increasing frequency until they were averaging about one per week. She had trouble with weight gain. The edema in her legs and feet started to return.

This was about the time that I was getting involved with Dr. Esselstyn's program. I explained the concept and benefits of a plant-based diet to her, but she was dubious. She hadn't read the books, I wasn't a doctor, and a prophet is rarely accepted in his own land.

A nugget of wisdom in Dr. Esselstyn's program prerequisites is that you must attend with a partner, preferably your spouse. Barb agreed to come only out of support, as my wife. But God bless Dr. Esselstyn. His thorough but concise explanations of twenty-five years of research won the day, for at the end of the program, during the question-and-answer time, a little hand rose from our corner of the room.

Barb told the group that although I was attending the program, she was the one who had had the heart attack. It was the first time she had ever fully understood the cause of the disease. The cause had finally been explained and the cure thrown in for good measure. On the way home that evening, she turned to me and said, "If we're going to do this thing right, we have to clean out the pantry." And we did! The nugget paid off; not only with her initial support, but with the support we continue to give each other.

Barb experienced the following changes in her condition:

- One angina attack a few days after program, and no angina attacks since.
- No further edema.
- She can wrestle on the floor with the grandkids.
- She lost 40-plus pounds and four dress sizes.

Sometimes she seems more excited about losing dress sizes than angina attacks, but after you don't have them for a while, you don't think about them anymore. It's just like how I no longer think about doing the basement stairs three steps at a time—I just do it.

The third part of the story is about my father. At eighty-seven, he has had two bypass surgeries and two pacemakers. As I said, with each of his bypass surgeries I saw a pronounced drop in his strength and cognitive skills. These were never more evident than before and after surgeries. Dad came to live with us after Mom passed away in January 2009. His condition at the time was:

- He'd been diagnosed with congestive heart failure.
- He could hardly get around. He shuffled more than walked. It was an effort to go back and forth from the kitchen to the bedroom.
- He didn't drive.

- He had frequent angina attacks.
- He was thin and very frail.
- He suffered from indigestion.
- He frequently took laxatives for constipation.
- He had type 2 diabetes and was taking oral medication for this.

By default, he ate the same as we did. He didn't like it and hated the "cow food" we ate. But he ate it. We observed the following changes in his condition:

- He slowly improved. His strength returned and he began a healthy weight gain.
- He could now stand to wash dishes without sit-down breaks.
- Because of consistent good blood sugar indications, his doctor took him off the diabetes medication. His diabetes was now being controlled by diet alone.
- He has fewer problems with constipation and indigestion.
- He began driving again.
- He's had no recent angina attacks.

I'd like to say that we are all living happily ever after. But there is one glitch. It is an important glitch. Dad improved so much and was feeling so good that he started leaving the house more often. Suddenly he had days when he just wasn't hungry. He had nausea and diarrhea, and the constipation returned.

It was only when we discovered the empty packages under his bed that we found out about his "departure" from our lifestyle. The dangerous glitch is that you start to feel so good that you go back. Dad had started buying junk food and sneaking it into his room. The good news is that he has sworn off cookie and cheese-curl binges and is feeling better again.

The New Menu

We are still fledgling vegans. I do still miss many of the old foods, but I don't miss angina, weakness, indigestion, high blood pressure, and 38-inch pants.

We learn more every day. We try new foods, new recipes. Some are miserable failures, many are delicious. We have retasted a couple of our old favorite foods since we switched to plant-based and found them incredibly greasy, full of salt, and almost unpalatable. So while I think I miss them, I know I really don't.

Barb makes a wonderful lentil soup in the pressure cooker. It's easy. Just chop up all of the constituent vegetables, throw in the lentils, add vegetable stock, seal the pot, and cook for a half hour. It's great coming out, but even better the next day.

I was never a lover of vegetables. Munching down a whole bowl of greens is tedious. One of the most effective ways I found to increase my intake of greens has been making green smoothies. My concoctions have a less than stellar aesthetic quality; mixing blueberries in with deep green kale, strawberries, lettuce, and a banana doesn't yield an eye pleaser. But they are antioxidant rich, loaded with fiber and vital nutrients. They taste good and make a great replacement for sugar-filled soda.

Philosophy

I have approached the whole thing with a two-part philosophy:

1. The thought that I can never have a certain food again is depressing, so I compromise and say I'm just not going to have that food today. I can't do forever, but I can do a day.
2. I ask myself, "Am I going to die if I *don't* eat this steak?" No. But I might die if I do.

The whole thing starts to sound like an AA meeting, and maybe it is; there is certainly an addictive quality about the diet of Western civilization. But I don't really mind being labeled as recovering fatty-food addicts.

My body tells me that I feel better. The documented studies say that at least some of the damage will heal. So I am encouraged. So it is good. So there is life after hamburger.

I really love Robert's attitude of willingness and levity; he takes it all seriously, but he has fun and gives himself a break. He has a good sense of humor and adventure, and he's leaning in to a healthier life—and bringing his family along with him—with gusto.

I highly recommend Dr. Esselstyn's book *Prevent and Reverse Heart Disease*; it's packed with stories like Robert's and is thoroughly substantiated by peer-reviewed research and hard science. Considering that the United States contains just 5 percent of the global population, but every year, physicians in American hospitals perform more than 50 percent of all the angioplasties and bypass procedures in the entire world, the information in those pages is highly relevant.

In his book, Dr. Esselstyn writes: "If you eat to save your heart . . . you gain protection from a host of other ailments that have been linked to dietary factors, including impotence and cancers of the breast, prostate, colon, rectum, uterus, ovaries. And if you are eating for good health in this way, here's a side benefit you might not have expected: for the rest of your life, you will never again have to count calories or worry about your weight." Here again, all upside.

Declawing Diabetes

One out of every three children born after the year 2000 will be diagnosed with type 2 diabetes. Can you believe that? One in three! What the heck is going on?

To understand diabetes better, and to learn how to reverse it, I spoke with Dr. Neal Barnard, whom you met earlier. He's an adjunct associate professor of medicine at the George Washington University School of Medicine, the author of numerous scientific articles in leading peer-reviewed journals, and a frequent lecturer at the American Diabetes Association's scientific sessions. His diabetes research was funded by the National Institutes of Health, the U.S. government's research branch. He is also the author of *Dr. Neal Barnard's Program for Reversing Diabetes*.

Straight from the Source:
Neal Barnard, MD, on Diabetes

KF: **Why is type 2 diabetes suddenly so prevalent?**
NB: Diets are changing, not just in the U.S., but worldwide. Diabetes seems to follow the spread of meaty, high-fat, high-calorie diets. In Japan, for example, the traditional rice-based diet kept the population generally healthy and thin for many centuries. Up until 1980, only 1 to 5 percent of Japanese adults over age forty had diabetes. Starting around that time, however, the rapid westernization of the diet meant that meat, milk, cheese, and sodas became fashionable. Waistlines expanded, and, by 1990, diabetes prevalence in Japan had climbed to 11 to 12 percent.

The same sort of trend has occurred in the U.S. Over the last century, per capita meat consumption increased from about 125 pounds per year (which was already very high compared with other countries) in the early 1900s to over 200 pounds today. In other words, the average American now eats 75 pounds more meat every year than the average American of a century ago. In the same interval, cheese intake soared from less than 4 pounds per person per year to about 33 pounds today. Sugar intake has gone up, too, by about 30 pounds per person per year. Where are we putting all that extra meat, cheese, and sugar? It contributes to body fat, of course, and diabetes follows. Today, about 13 percent of the

U.S. adult population has type 2 diabetes, although many of them are not yet aware they have it.

KF: What causes diabetes?
NB: Normally, the cells of the body use the simple sugar glucose as fuel, the way a car uses gasoline. Glucose comes from starchy or sweet foods we eat, and the hormone insulin escorts it into the muscle cells to power our movements. Glucose also passes into our brain cells to power our thoughts. In type 2 diabetes, the cells resist insulin's action, so glucose has trouble getting into the cells.

KF: What happens to the body when a person develops diabetes? What's the fallout?
NB: If glucose can't get into the cells, it builds up in the blood. It is as if gasoline coming out of a gas pump somehow can't get into your gas tank, and it ends up spilling over the side of your car, coming in through your car windows, and dribbling all over the pavement. It is a dangerous situation. The abnormally high levels of glucose circulating in the bloodstream are toxic to the blood vessels, especially the tiny blood vessels of the eyes, the kidneys, the extremities, and the heart.

KF: Is it really that serious, or can we just take a drug for it?
NB: A person with diabetes loses more than a decade of life, on average; about three-quarters will die prematurely of a heart attack. It is also a leading cause of blindness, amputations, and loss of kidney function. Many drugs are available, from insulin to oral medications and an ever-increasing va-

riety of other medications. In order to protect the heart, many patients are also put on medications to lower cholesterol and blood pressure. And yet these medications only slow the progression of the disease; many people have serious complications despite being on medications.

Let me emphasize that this grim scenario does not have to occur. If an unhealthy diet is the cause, a better diet can provide the answer to this problem.

KF: How can we avoid it?
NB: The key is to help our body's insulin to work normally. So long as your body's insulin can escort glucose into the cells normally, diabetes will not occur. The resistance to insulin that leads to diabetes appears to be caused by a buildup of fat inside the muscle cells and also inside the liver. Let me draw an analogy: I arrive home from work one day and put my key in my front door lock. But I notice the key does not turn properly, and the door does not open. Peering inside the lock, I see that someone has jammed chewing gum into the lock. Now, if the insulin "key" cannot open up the cell to glucose, there is something interfering with it. It's not chewing gum, of course. The problem is fat. In the same way that chewing gum in a lock makes it hard to open your front door, fat particles inside muscle cells interfere with insulin's efforts to open the cell to glucose. This fat comes from beef, chicken, fish, cooking oils, dairy products, etc. The answer is to avoid these fatty foods. People who avoid all animal products obviously get no animal fat at all, they appear to have much less fat buildup inside their cells, and their risk of diabetes is extremely low. Minimizing oils helps, too.

And we can go beyond prevention. When people who already have diabetes adopt a low-fat vegan diet, their condition often improves dramatically. In our research, funded by the U.S. government, we found that a vegan diet is more effective than the current traditional diabetes diet, and is much safer than a low-carb diet.

"When people who already have diabetes adopt a low-fat vegan diet, their condition often improves dramatically."—Dr. Neal Barnard

---

KF: What about the claim that a vegetarian diet has too many starches, which raises blood sugar?
NB: Starchy foods, such as whole grains, beans, and vegetables, are healthful foods, and the body is designed to use the glucose that they hold. In type 2 diabetes, the body has lost some of this ability. But the answer is not to avoid starches but to restore the body's ability to use them. After all, cultures whose diets are traditionally high in carbohydrate—Japan, China, Latin America—have had very low diabetes rates until meat, cheese, and other fatty foods displace their healthy carbohydrate-rich diets; only then does diabetes become more common.

The Atkins fad unfortunately left many people imagining that carbohydrate (that is, starch) is somehow risky. That notion is as unscientific as suggesting that water or oxygen is dangerous. The body needs all these things for good health.

A similarly persistent but misguided idea is the blood-type diet approach. A popular book on this subject said that people with type A blood should follow a vegetarian diet but that people with type O blood should not. Unfortunately many readers with type O blood followed this advice, which turned out to be quite wrong. The fact is, people with type O blood do as well as everyone else on a plant-based diet. A vegan diet is helpful and effective, regardless of blood type.

KF: Let me diverge for just a moment and ask you about soy, since it seems to be a hot-button issue. The word on the street is that soy products can have hormonal effects. If a woman is at high risk for breast cancer, is soy a bad idea?
NB: Many studies have looked at this question, and the results are consistent. Women who include soy products in their routine are less likely than other women to develop breast cancer. In January 2008, researchers at the University of Southern California quantified the benefit on the basis of the most rigorously controlled studies to date: Women averaging one cup of soy milk or about one-half cup of tofu daily have about a 30 percent lower risk of developing breast cancer, compared with women who have little or no soy products in their diets.

KF: But what about the hormones? I've heard it said that soy acts like estrogen in the body and adds to problems like girls starting their periods too soon and the development of certain types of cancers?
NB: It is true that there are hormones in soy products. The phytoestrogens found in soybeans (*phyto* means "plant") are

much weaker than the estrogens (female sex hormones) in a woman's bloodstream. One common explanation for soy's beneficial effects is that phytoestrogens reduce the effects of a woman's natural estrogens. Think of the estrogens in a woman's body as a fleet of jumbo jets. They land at an airport and pull up to the jetways where they will discharge their passengers and baggage. But what if the jetways were already occupied by small private planes? The jumbo jets would be unable to dock, and would be left sitting idle on the tarmac.

When phytoestrogens attach to the estrogen receptors on cells, they are like little private planes. They partially block a woman's natural estrogens from attaching. From a health standpoint, that's good. Many women have too much estrogen in their blood. And since estrogens tend to fuel the growth of cancer cells, anything that reduces estrogen effects helps cut cancer risk.

But recent research has shown that this explanation is almost certainly inadequate; soy's effects are much more complicated, but it illustrates how foods can temper the negative effects of hormones.

KF: Does soy increase your risk of fibroids?

NB: It might even reduce the risk. Fibroids are knots of muscle tissue that form within the thin muscle layer that lies beneath the uterine lining. Estrogens can encourage these muscle cells to overgrow. Fibroids are not cancerous, but sometimes they become large and painful.

A study of Japanese women found that the more soy women ate, the less likely they were to need a hysterectomy, suggesting that fibroids were less frequent. In a study of women in Washington State, soy did not seem to help or hurt, perhaps because American women eat very little soy, compared with their Japanese counterparts. What did have a big effect in this study were lignans, a group of phyto-estrogens found in flaxseed and whole grains. The women consuming the highest amounts of these foods had less than half the risk of fibroids, compared with the women who generally skipped these foods. So, again, phytoestrogens seem beneficial, countering the effects of a woman's natural estrogens, although in this case the benefit comes from foods other than soy.

***KF*: What if you have hypothyroidism?**
***NB*:** Some studies have suggested that soy isoflavones take up some of the iodine that would normally be used to make thyroid hormone. The same is true of fiber supplements and some medications. In theory, then, people who consume soy might need slightly more iodine in their diets (iodine is found in many plant foods, and especially in seaweed and iodized salt). However, clinical studies show that soy products do not cause hypothyroidism.

Soy products do seem to reduce the absorption of medicines used to treat hypothyroidism. If you take these medicines, your health-care provider can easily check to see if your dose needs to be adjusted.

***KF*: Okay; back to diabetes; can it be reversed?**
***NB*:** Yes. When people begin a healthful diet, most see big improvements in weight, cholesterol, and their blood sugar.

Their need for medications diminishes, and some may not need medications at all. In some cases, you would never know they had had diabetes. However, I caution people not to simply throw their medications away. They need to speak with their doctors so they can alter their medication regimens only when and if it is appropriate.

Let me describe a case: A man named Vance joined our study. His father was dead by age thirty, and Vance was thirty-one when he was diagnosed with diabetes. As our study began, he started a low-fat, vegan diet and gradually lost about 60 pounds over a year's time. His blood sugar control returned to normal, and his doctor discontinued his medications. Imagine what it feels like to see family members assaulted by this disease, but then to realize that you have effectively tackled it by making healthful adjustments to your diet.

Vance also encouraged me to mention that it is not only blood sugar that gets better; his erectile dysfunction also improved dramatically, too—in case anyone needs an extra motivator.

Ha! I love that last comment! And that was a result, by the way, of Vance's circulation being improved (more on that in the next chapter). My takeaway here is that diabetes is deeply connected to having too much fat in the body, and that fat is largely a result of eating meat and dairy. What is so exciting is that you can really reverse this disease, and you can do it in a fairly short amount of time.

As informative as this talk with the doctor has been, there is nothing so compelling as a personal story, so here is Natala Constantine's.

Natala Constantine's Story:
Her Diabetes Cure

I was diagnosed with diabetes two weeks after my husband and I got married. I was twenty-five years old. I sat in a doctor's office, trying to remain calm as the doctors and nurses spoke to me, telling me that my blood sugar was dangerously high. My husband and I sat in an emergency room listening to a doctor explain how my blood had turned acidic, how I was fortunate to be alive, how they were not sure if I would make it. I survived that night, only to spend many nights wishing that I hadn't.

I spent five years of my life trying everything to control my diabetes. I went to doctor after doctor, all of whom put me on different cocktails of drugs. Some would work for a time, but in the end, I was constantly adjusting the medications, constantly battling high blood sugar, and still battling high cholesterol, being morbidly obese, hormonal problems, blood pressure issues, nerve damage, early arthritis, and other physical problems, mostly caused from diabetes.

My story is like millions of others. I tried everything—every diet, every workout regimen, and every drug. I was on what doctors would prescribe as a "healthy diet," which always meant lots of animal protein and almost no carbohydrates, including vegetables. I was told that a high–animal protein diet was the only way to control my diabetes. My blood sugar would improve at times, but I could never decrease my medicines, and my health overall was deteriorating.

When I turned thirty, my diabetes remained out of control. I was still on the doctor-prescribed diet, high in animal proteins. My weight tipped the scale at the time at over 360 pounds. I was in the gym two to three hours a day and I was losing only a couple of pounds a month. Then I developed an infection in my lower right calf.

For a diabetic, an infection anywhere in the foot area or lower leg is dangerous. I already had significant nerve damage to my lower legs due to poor circulation. I already had severe pain in my feet, caused by early arthritis in the bones in the tops of my feet. And now I was facing an infection in my leg.

The doctor looked at my leg and expressed grave concern that the infection wasn't healing. She told me that if things didn't improve, I might be facing partial amputation.

I was devastated. I was only thirty. I didn't think things like this happened until later in life. I thought about my husband and how this seemed so unfair to him. Our life together was completely focused on my illness. I sat in the doctor's office and sobbed. I was on nine different medications, I had no energy to work, I was trying everything that I was told to do, and nothing helped.

I got to the point where I questioned if I had the strength to go on. I would cry myself to sleep at night. I didn't want to continue living life as a morbidly obese, out-of-control diabetic. But I realized that I did want to live.

On one of the darkest days, a good friend suggested that I look at a natural approach to my diabetes. She told me that I needed to look at food as medicine.

I was angry with her at first. How dare she suggest something so simple? Didn't she know that I had been to the best doctors? That I was on the best medications? That I was injecting myself with insulin, that I was on the best diet, that I was working out?

But I did take her advice to heart. I started searching for new answers and came across a few books that talked about healing diabetes naturally. I had always been completely against the idea of doing anything "natural." I thought the approach was absurd. As I read, though, I couldn't ignore the facts or the science. So many of the books described my situation exactly.

I decided to stop doing what was not working and to try something completely different.

My reading led me to a 100 percent healthy plant-based diet. After years of eating all that meat, I decided to make the leap.

For the first three weeks I felt as though I was ridding myself of much more than animal products. I realized that I had many powerful addictions to food. Food had a hold on me that I could not even conceptualize prior to those three weeks. I would sit in my car and cry outside of sub shops, just wanting a tuna melt.

Before that first three weeks I was on over 100 units of insulin per day, and in three weeks I was taking no insulin.

In about a month, I was once again in my doctor's office, watching as they looked at my numbers in utter amazement. When they asked me what I did, I told them I had adopted a completely plant-based diet. They didn't seem surprised at all and told me that plant-based diets were helping to reverse diabetes. When I asked why they had not suggested it, they told me "because it is not practical."

There I was, morbidly obese, taking nine drugs, shooting insulin into myself multiple times per day, suffering nerve damage and severe pain, and yet they thought that changing my diet in a fairly easy way would be less practical?

It was at that moment that I took my health into my own hands. I found out everything I possibly could about plant-based nutrition. I learned everything I could about how my body works and which foods were meant to go into my body and which foods never were.

Everything changed from that moment. I slowly decreased all the other diabetes medicines I was on. I lowered my cholesterol without drugs, I lowered my blood pressure without drugs, I corrected my hormonal problems without drugs. And that infection on my leg? It completely healed. The arthritis in my feet? It went away.

After years of battling with the scale, the weight finally started to come off. I've lost a total of 160 pounds. While still obese, with over 100 pounds left to lose, for the first time in my life, I can see the light at the end of a very dark tunnel.

Today, I am medicine free. I have been on a complete plant-based diet for a little more than a year. This journey took me to places I would have never imagined. It took me to a place beyond myself. When I became aware of my body and what I was feeding it, my life changed. For years, I consumed death, and for that I almost lost my life. The way I lived my life, the way I looked at foods, was such that I was not an active participant in my life. I was not living, I was barely surviving. I was not experiencing life, I was going through motions, hoping that someday someone would find a magical cure.

It wasn't until I discovered that I was the key to my health that my life completely changed. Today I live with hope. I live with knowing that I am in complete control of my health and preventable disease. I live with knowing that I cannot rely on anyone except myself to make conscious choices every single day that either give life or take life away. Once I let go and made the decision to live, my life changed completely.

Today, both my husband and I live and thrive on a complete plant-based diet. Our lives have become filled with hope. We thrive, and we continue to learn.

There is an answer to type 2 diabetes, an answer that is found not in a doctor's office or pharmaceutical lab, but in our gardens. Today, I am living a life free of pain, free of harsh drugs, and free of out-of-control diabetes.

Cancer, heart disease, diabetes: If changing to a plant-based diet can halt or reverse the course of these "killer" diseases, imagine what it can do for you if you are not even ill. It can put you on a course that is life changing. I have heard it said that adopting a plant-based diet is "too extreme." I like Dr. Ornish's retort, which is something like this: So changing your diet is extreme, but triple bypass surgery and a lifetime on cholesterol-lowering drugs, that's conservative? Amazingly, in the eyes of the mainstream medical community, the answer is yes.

You may be thinking that a vegan diet may be too challenging, and a more moderate diet change may seem more sensible. I always encourage people to "lean in" to a diet change so that the changes come comfortably and gradually. But when you have specific health concerns, a moderate change might not do the trick. If you are at serious risk it makes good sense to intervene in a major way. After all, if you were using medicines, you would not prescribe cold medicine for heart disease or cancer; you would prescribe the most effective medications in the best regimen possible. The same is true for diet. Someone who is killing himself with food needs a major change.

Interestingly enough, lots of research shows that the more changes people are asked to make, the more they make. Perhaps it's more exciting to do a lifestyle overhaul rather than to just pick and choose a few small changes. It might not stick the first time you try, but just like quitting smoking or achieving any new skill, you may need more than one try.

I have devoted a section at the back of this book to "making the switch." It's full of ideas for what to buy, how to plan meals, and good snack foods. Do hang out in that section of the book for a while; I think you will find some interesting meal choices and tips. Most important of all, be gentle and kind with yourself. Try it, and try it, and try it until it sticks. Lean, and if you are so moved, leap!

PROMISE 3:

You Will Live longer— and Better

Did you know?

- The current generation of children just might be the first to have shorter life expectancies than their parents, reversing the trend of ever-longer lives.
- The poor circulation from clogged arteries that can cause heart disease and stroke can also cause impotence and dementia. For the same reason that a vegan diet can reverse heart disease, it can also improve brain and sexual health.
- Whole plant-based foods have antiaging and anti-disease properties animal foods do not.

Modern culture has a love affair with meat. It's everywhere—in the vast majority of homes and in most menu

items. You look at the commercials on TV and you are per-
suaded to believe it's wholesome, natural, and good for you.
It also looks fun and social to enjoy meaty, cheesy dishes with
friends and family. To many, meat signifies prosperity—not
too long ago, only those of generous means could afford to eat
meat regularly. But it's become obvious over the past few
decades that this prosperity, and the constant availability of
food that comes along with it, is actually harming our health.
We've already looked at the effects of our expanding waistlines on our health, but there's an even more sinister aspect
of our prosperity diets: the fact that they're shortening our
lives and dramatically diminishing our quality of life as we
age. In fact, the current generation of children just might be
the first to have shorter life expectancies than their parents,
reversing the trend of ever-longer lives.

The CDC (Centers for Disease Control and Prevention)
lists the top three U.S. causes of death in 2006 as heart disease (631,636), cancer (559,888), and stroke (137,119). Just
a couple of spots down on the list, diabetes killed 72,449.

We've already examined the fact that these causes of
death can be inextricably linked to our diets—and that eating a more plant-based diet may actually reverse heart disease and stroke, and lower your cancer and diabetes risks
substantially. So, of course, these simple effects will all but
guarantee you a longer life (well, unless your newfound vitality turns you into another Evel Knievel!).

Quality of Life

Longevity isn't just about living longer, of course—it's about
being healthy and living better, right through our twilight

years. We want to feel vibrant and full of energy; we want to grow old with the physical and mental vitality to enjoy every minute we have on earth. After all, who wants to live a few extra years if it means being in constant pain or going senile?

People today might be living longer, but in our culture, they are also spending more time suffering from chronic diseases that cause weakness or incapacity (physical and mental). And, of course, just as our diet can kill us from heart disease or cancer, it can also incapacitate us and make our lives less pleasant (or even excruciating) from seriously debilitating conditions like dementia or Alzheimer's, or less-serious warning signs of bigger problems like impotence, lethargy, and bad circulation.

According to the CDC, the life span of the average American in 2006 (the most recent numbers available) was 77.7 years, which is similar to other developed countries. Nearly 78 years of life sounds pretty good—after all, it's far more than most people could expect just a hundred years ago—until we take a look at some of the problems that more and more of us are suffering through as we age.

Since I started writing about moving toward a plant-based diet, one thing that I hear from people—constantly—is that their change in diet has dramatically improved their life, almost instantly. Once people eliminate animal products from their diet and replace them with whole grains and legumes, their body can digest their food more easily. They feel lighter, have more energy, need less sleep and coffee, and so on. This only makes sense: Any food that can clog your arteries and kill you from heart disease, or lead to cancer, obesity, and diabetes, is sure to have serious short-term consequences as well (e.g., obesity or angina, and the many quality-of-life effects associated with both conditions).

Of course, the properties of whole vegan foods—fiber, complex carbohydrates, healthy plant proteins—are exactly what everyone in the medical establishment tells us we should eat more of. And the nutrients inherent in animal foods—animal proteins, saturated fat—are the nutrients that, over the long term, make us sick and can kill us. Again, animal products have no fiber at all, and no carbohydrates of any kind. That's a prescription for ill health, and the more of them you eat, the less healthy you are likely to be.

Dr. Dean Ornish explains that "whole foods such as fruits, vegetables, grains, and beans contain literally thousands of other substances that are protective, having antiaging, anti-cancer, and anti–heart disease properties. These include fiber, isoflavones, carotenoids, bioflavonoids, retinols, lycopene, genistein, on and on." He talks about the fact that when people adopt his low-fat plant-based diet to lose weight or reverse their heart disease, their sexual function, mental clarity, and energy all improve as well. As he puts it, they adopt the diet because they "fear dying." Very soon, they see dramatic positive results, and they stay on the diet because they enjoy living.

Let's talk about just two of the benefits of a plant-based diet, for your long-term joy in living: prevention of dementia and impotence.

Alzheimer's and Other Forms of Dementia

Alzheimer's disease, which affects more than 5 million people in the United States alone, is an irreversible degenerative brain disease that has to be, I think, the worst "natural" way to die. You lose your memory, your personality changes, you basically become a different (and certainly not better) person—an infant in your old age. And then you die—Alzheimer's is the sixth most common cause of death in the United States, and it's growing in prevalence (by more than 40 percent from 2000 to 2006, according to the Alzheimer's Association).

Not surprisingly, the causes of Alzheimer's and other forms of dementia are the same as the causes of heart disease. According to a 2010 report from the Alzheimer's Association, "A growing body of evidence suggests that the health of the brain—one of the body's most highly vascular organs—is closely linked to the overall health of the heart and blood vessels." The Association specifically notes that Alzheimer's and other forms of dementia have the same risk factors as "high cholesterol, type 2 diabetes, high blood pressure, smoking, obesity and physical inactivity. . . . Many of these risk factors are modifiable—that is, they can be changed to decrease the likelihood of developing both cardiovascular disease and the cognitive decline associated with Alzheimer's and other forms of dementia."

"The link between heart disease and Alzheimer's disease is growing in strength every few months," according to the Association's scientific director, Bill Thies, speaking to *ABC World News*. "And we predict it will continue to grow. . . . I'm not surprised that there's a relationship. . . . The heart is the organ that supplies essential elements to many parts of the body, and the brain is just one of the first."

So we can easily make connections based on our analysis of heart disease, obesity, and diabetes. For the same reason that almost 100 percent of heart disease is preventable, dementia—including Alzheimer's—can be staved off by a healthy vegan diet. And sure enough, we learn from Dr. Esselstyn that "at least half of all senile mental impairment is caused by vascular injury to the brain" and that "clogged arteries serving the brain and clogged arteries serving the heart are part and parcel of the same disease."

He tells of one study of 500 eighty-five-year-olds, which found that fully one-third of them showed some form of dementia. A careful analysis revealed that in half of those with dementia, their mental impairment was due to a diseased arterial blood supply to the brain. Similarly, a study in the Netherlands focused on 5,000 people between the ages of fifty-five and ninety-four. "The researchers studied the circulation in the brains of all their subjects, then asked them to perform various written tests of mental acuity. The results were quite clear: those suffering from artery disease and thus impaired circulation in the brain performed less well on the tests than did those whose arteries were clean. Age made no difference. Arterial health was the variable that counted."

Dr. Esselstyn concludes, "Just as you are not doomed to heart disease as you grow older, you also are not doomed to mental deterioration. Most cases of stroke and dementia, like heart disease, need never occur. Your aorta, along with all your other arteries, can be as clean at ninety years of age as they were when you were nine."

Wow.

And Now Impotence

Viagra is the best-selling drug in U.S. history, but apparently it needn't be so. Once upon a time, doctors thought that impotence was a purely mental condition. Now we know that the vast majority of cases are physical. And the cause of impotence: clogged arteries.

You might have read about the links between obesity and impotence, and diabetes and impotence. Of course, overweight men and women have worse circulation than people who maintain a healthy weight. One study published by the American Urological Association found that obese men had twice the impotence rates of men of a healthy weight. Similarly, the Harvard Medical School explains that "diabetes can cause nerve and artery damage in the genital area, disrupting the blood flow necessary for an erection."

Impotence can also be a sign in itself of other problems. Dr. Esselstyn and Dr. Ornish have both written about the connection between impotence and elevated cholesterol. According to Esselstyn, impotence is "as robust a predictor of cardiovascular disease as elevated cholesterol, smoking, or a strong family history of the disease." Dr. Ornish writes in the introduction to his book *Eat More, Weigh Less*: "When you get less blood flow to your sexual organs, your sexual potency decreases . . . The reason that Viagra is one of the best-selling drugs of all time is that so many people need it. Impotence . . . is a silent epidemic, present in at least one-half of men over the age of forty. Did you know you're much more likely to be impotent if your cholesterol level is elevated?"

I am talking here about impotence, a male problem, but for women, too, sexual pleasure is also dependent on blood flow. So although women don't experience impotence, clogged arteries can—for the exact same reason they inhibit erectile function in men—inhibit sexual pleasure for women.

A Few Case Studies on Plant-based Diet and Circulation

I have included a variety of case studies in this book—anecdotes that support the overwhelming scientific evidence that diet can be used to beat back the greatest health scourges that are affecting the developed nations. When I started looking for stories, I was bowled over by how many there are—including dozens in Dr. Esselstyn's book, and many more on Dr. John McDougall's website (more on him soon). And they are all so deeply inspiring. In a moment, I'm going to introduce you to Dr. Ruth Heidrich, who is one of my heroes, but first, I'd like to mention just a few from two of my favorite nutritional experts.

Dr. Esselstyn explains:

> In 1996, I used plant-based nutrition to aggressively reduce the risk factors in a patient with demonstrably poor circulation to a portion of heart muscle. A cardiac PET scan noted the problem just prior to my intervention. Within ten days of her starting a plant-based diet and a low dose of cholesterol-lowering drug, the patient's cholesterol level fell from 248 mg/dL to 137. After just three weeks of therapy, a repeat scan showed restored circulation to the area

of heart muscle that had been deprived. There was no doubt what had happened: a profound change in lifestyle, adopting strictly plant-based nutrition, brought about a rapid restoration of the endothelial cells' capacity to manufacture nitric oxide, and that, in turn, restored circulation.

Esselstyn tells of a man who came to him with multiple blockages in his coronary arteries. He was experiencing chest pain when he walked, and was scheduled for bypass surgery. After just eleven days on a low-fat, plant-based diet, the pain was gone. He canceled his surgery. In addition to publishing his best-selling book, Dr. Esselstyn also published his findings in the *American Journal of Cardiology*.

Dr. Ornish tells of "a man named Mark [who] came to my office and showed me a photograph of how he looked two years earlier. I hardly recognized him—because he weighed 335 pounds then and only 165 pounds now. He lost 170 pounds by following the program outlined in *Eat More, Weigh Less* and has not regained it."

Of course, anecdotes are not science; but these doctors—and others—have published their results, which prove that these anecdotes put faces to the vast numbers of people who have beaten heart disease, cancer, diabetes, obesity, impotence, dementia, and more—by changing the way they eat.

Dr. Caldwell Esselstyn, Dr. T. Colin Campbell, Dr. Dean Ornish, and Dr. Neal Barnard agree that a whole-foods, plant-based diet minimizes the likelihood of stroke, obesity, hypertension, type 2 diabetes, and cancers of the breast, prostate, colon, rectum, uterus, and ovary.

Other Factors That Influence Longevity

Okay, just so you don't think I'm *only* about a plant-based diet, here are some other recommendations for long-term health and happiness!

1. Regular physical activity

It's no secret that regular exercise benefits the body in a wide variety of ways. Regular physical activity helps us look better, increases energy levels, and boosts self-confidence. Evidence also suggests that it may help you live longer. Moderate physical activity is associated with a lower risk of heart disease and diabetes. A 2005 study conducted by the U.S. Department of Public Health and the Erasmus University Medical Center in Rotterdam found that women over fifty gained 1.5 years of life if they were moderately active, and 3.5 years if they led highly physically active lifestyles. While it is difficult with our superbusy lifestyles to be physically active, it is not impossible. It may be just a matter of trading up your morning coffee routine for a quick jog or brisk walk around the neighborhood that could make a huge difference in the length and quality of your life!

2. Not smoking

If you're not a smoker, congratulate yourself on avoiding a particularly strong risk factor associated with a reduced life span. If you are a smoker, or are in the process of trying to quit, realize that becoming an ex-smoker is one of the best things you can do to extend your life. Researchers at the University of Bristol in England found that each cigarette reduces your life by eleven minutes. Huge bodies of well-established research have conclusively proven the direct link between mortality and smoking. The 1998 book *Dying to Quit*, by Dr. Janet Brigham, a specialist in the effects of tobacco, estimates that a typical smoker may lose as many as twenty-five years of life. Clearly, quitting smoking drastically extends your life, benefitting you and your loved ones.

3. Avoiding (and learning to manage) stress

Stress is yet another aspect of life that, if excessive, can rob you of months or years. Not all stress is bad—in fact, some stress is actually positive and normal. But being constantly stressed means that your nervous system is always on alert, and that is detrimental to your heart, your immune system, and your overall health. Meditate, take walks, talk things through with trusted friends and advisers. Just breathe, and put one foot in front of the other; you will get through.

4. Limiting alcohol consumption

The news on alcohol seems conflicting these days, with one study telling us that a glass of red wine a day may promote health, and others saying that any alcohol is detrimental. What these studies agree on, however, is that anything more than moderate consumption of alcohol decreases our longevity. In women, this may be especially true, as we metabolize alcohol at a slower rate than men do. The CDC suggests that for women moderate drinking is no more than one drink per day, for men no more than two.

Too much alcohol intake is correlated with many destructive things: an increased risk of accidents and/or unintended injuries, cirrhosis of the liver, high blood pressure, and some cancers, including liver, mouth, throat, larynx, and esophageal cancers.

Conclusion

As we've seen, it's harder to find a common deadly disease that *isn't* linked in some way to diet. With the abundance of advice out there on extending your life, it's easy to be confused. But consider that a plant-based diet is so clearly linked to a better and longer life that even the American Dietetic Association, which requires overwhelming scientific evidence, has endorsed it as helping to reduce risks for heart disease, cancer, diabetes, and obesity. Adopting a whole new, plant-based set of rules for eating could be one of the most dramatic, life-extending changes you'll ever make. As Dr. Ornish explains, "I find it gratifying to know that when people make the diet and lifestyle changes I recommend, they not only lose weight but also improve their health and well-being."

And now, the story of one of my heroes.

Ruth Heidrich, PhD, is the very definition of living long and well. At seventy-five years old, she has been running every day for more than forty years, and has been a vegan for almost thirty years. She credits her veganism both for her formidable intellect—she has her bachelor's and master's degrees in psychology, her PhD in health education, and has lectured across the country, from Stanford to Cornell—and for her excellent health. She has won eight gold medals in the Senior Olympics, has completed six Ironman Triathlons, and has set age-group records in every distance from the 100-meter dash to the 5K road race to ultramarathon, pentathlon, and triathlon.

Ruth Heidrich's Story:
You Can Be Fit at Any Age

My awakening to the harm of dairy and meat came in middle age, almost thirty years ago. I was forty-seven years old and healthy—or so I thought. Like so many athletes of my generation, I ate lots of chicken, fish, and low-fat dairy.

While in the shower one morning, I found a lump in my right breast. My doctor thought cancer unlikely, but scheduled a mammogram, to rule it out, he said. I was, as you can imagine, delighted when the results came back negative; to be safe, I was encouraged to schedule annual mammograms, which I did. For the next two years, the results were negative.

That third year, though, my life was turned upside down: positive. And not just positive, but the lump was now golf-ball size. The doctor did an immediate excisional biopsy (meaning that he intended to remove the entire lump) and found that it was infiltrating ductal cancer, an invasive cancer that was already spreading to my bones, liver, and left lung. And because there were no clear margins, meaning they didn't get it all, I had to go back for more surgery.

My doctor, as well as other doctors I consulted, recommended standard cancer care—chemotherapy, radiation, tamoxifen. I wanted answers, but all I had were questions and uncertainty. No one could tell me if I had months to live, or years. They couldn't tell me if I might send the cancer into remission, or anything else. I felt totally powerless.

And even more: I felt betrayed. I was an athlete. I stayed away from high-fat foods and junk food. I ate a lot of chicken, fish, and low-fat dairy. How could this happen to me?

As I pondered chemotherapy, radiation, and so on—I got more and more scared. I read that people on chemotherapy didn't necessarily live for longer than people who didn't have chemotherapy. But by then I had resigned myself to it.

By the wildest of coincidences, I came across an advertisement for a research study that Dr. John Mc-Dougall was conducting with breast cancer patients. My first consultation with Dr. McDougall was revelatory. I'll never forget the first thing he said to me after he reviewed my record—that my cholesterol level of 236 put me at a risk of heart attack that was on par with my risk of dying from my cancer.

Dr. McDougall encouraged me to change my diet, noting that ample research had shown (and the evidence is much stronger now) that diet is linked to heart disease, cancer, diabetes, and a host of other ailments. In fact, making the dietary change was a condition of my being a subject in his study. Remarkably to me as one who grew up with "the four food groups," his biggest recommendation was the elimination of animal products, which constituted two of the four groups (and about half of what I was eating).

Once Dr. McDougall showed me the science, and explained the power of the research—especially about diet and cholesterol level—I was convinced. I adopted a vegan diet—and became a subject in his research study—that very day.

I know that some people find a vegan diet difficult to follow, but I can't understand how or why. For me, the diet opened me up to a range of foods that I had previously ignored. My old diet was centered on four animals, with everything else only making up "sides," that now strikes me as narrow and boring. My new vegan diet was exciting, colorful, and much more varied than my previous diet.

Anyway, my body responded immediately. And I do mean immediately: From that point on, I've had daily bowel movements—I had been constipated my entire life and had no idea why. Doctors had told me that going three or four times per week is normal for some people; maybe in a meat-based culture, but once you adopt a vegan diet and begin to go every day (sometimes repeatedly, especially if you're athletic and thus eat a lot), you realize that for the entirety of your pre-vegan life, you've been incubating rotting food for days at a time. You felt lethargic, heavy—and didn't even know why.

My oncologist assured me that my diet and cancer were unrelated, but I'd seen so much evidence linking diet and cancer that I didn't think he could possibly be correct. Since that time, I've read much more, studied the evidence, and I now understand that chicken and fish are at least as carcinogenic as beef and pork; they have more animal protein than beef and pork, and animal protein is the key carcinogenic agent, as anyone who has read Dr. T. Colin Campbell's work will understand.

Remarkably, the cancer had reversed and stopped growing, and my excruciating bone pain went away. It's been twenty-eight years, and I have not experienced another cancer flare-up. My reading of T. Colin Campbell's work convinces me that my diet stopped my cancer. I have no other explanation—and neither did my oncologist.

I can't remember how and when, but as I was going through the emotional and physical turmoil of grappling with cancer, I happened to see the Ironman Triathlon on television. I can't recall just what my thinking was—looking back on it, I can't begin to understand why I thought this would be a good idea—but somehow, I decided I had to do it. I'd been an athlete up until this time, and I knew I could handle the running. So really, I thought, why not tack on a 2.4 mile swim and 112-mile bike ride?

Obviously, my cancer and cholesterol level gave me pause. And my age gave me even more pause—

could a late-forties cancer survivor really complete this ultratriathlon, said to be one of the most grueling races in the world, done only by crazies? But I'd been devouring information on diet and health, and I was convinced that a vegan diet was the healthiest one imaginable, and that it would power me through. Regardless, I wanted to try; if it worked, I'd be able to tell everyone I met that my diet not only beat back my cancer, but it gave me the energy to compete in one of the toughest imaginable physical endeavors.

Since my diagnosis in 1982, I have completed the Ironman event six times, setting age-group records in the process. I've run sixty-seven marathons, and I've won nearly 1,000 gold medals (including eight in the Senior Olympics). And I've been declared by *Living Fit* magazine to be "one of the ten fittest women in North America." I have a fitness age of thirty-two.

In addition to the fact that I feel spectacular and have boundless energy on my vegan diet, I also want to briefly discuss osteoporosis. I have a history of this bone-degenerating disease on both sides of my family, so I've paid attention to it. What I have learned from the scientific studies is that the best way to prevent osteoporosis—by far—is to exercise. I wasn't surprised to learn, but am pleased to say that from the age of forty-seven to age sixty-four, my bone density increased significantly with each test—it's because of all the exercise I get.

Additionally, the arthritis that developed in my thirties vanished, and I was able to stop taking Naprosyn, the drug that doctors told me I'd be taking for the rest of my life. My joints today not only are not arthritic, but I actually do my own daily mini-triathlon as part of my regular training.

As someone who is so deeply convinced both that bad diets can kill us and that good diets can keep us healthy, I've been dispirited by the deafening silence of the medical community to the overwhelming scientific evidence in support of the work of Dr. McDougall, Dr. Esselstyn, Dr. Campbell, and others. I am pleased that Dr. Mehmet Oz has become famous preaching the diet gospel, but the information has yet to get to the masses.

And that's why I tell my story to everyone who will listen—because I think that if the world understood the link between diet and health, as well as how tasty and exciting vegan eating can be, there would be a food revolution . . . tomorrow.

You might want to check out some of Dr. John McDougall's best-selling books; they are extremely helpful and informative. He's a physician whose focus is healing the body through vegetarian cuisine, and he has many success stories that support his research. Dr. McDougall also has a ten-day residential program designed to turn your health around and give you a new program for eating and living. I highly recommend checking out his website for more information: www.drmcdougall.com.

You Will Take Yourself Out of Harm's Way

Did you know?

- All food poisoning—all foodborne viruses, bacteria, and antibiotic-resistant infections—comes from animals, including humans. (Yes, even the bacteria carried on spinach and tomatoes. See below.)
- Over 95 percent of the meat, dairy, and eggs we eat comes from factory farms, where the animals are pumped full of drugs to keep them alive and to speed up their development and productivity. In fact, chickens get twice the antibiotic dosing that cattle do, because the conditions they are raised in are the worst of the worst and therefore require more medicine just to keep them alive long enough to be killed for their meat.
- On average, the immune cells of vegetarians are twice as effective at destroying their targets—

not only cancer cells, but virus-infected cells as well—as the immune cells of meat eaters.

- In 2010, the Centers for Disease Control reported finding fecal contamination in 90 percent of poultry, 75 percent of beef, and 43 percent of the pork.

- Dairy cow and pig factories routinely dump millions of gallons of putrefying waste into massive open-air cesspits, which can then contaminate the water used to irrigate our crops. That's how a deadly fecal pathogen like *E. coli* O157:H7 can end up contaminating our spinach.

I recently came across this truly shocking fact: More people per year die from antibiotic-resistant infections than from prostate and breast cancer combined. And the numbers are going up at an alarming rate.

Why? Why have so many infections become resistant to drugs? Because factory farms are breeding grounds for ever more sophisticated bacteria. And why is that? Because when you try to keep animals in horrifically cramped conditions, literally living in their own waste, they are extremely susceptible to germs, so you have to dose them prophylactically (preventively) with antibiotics to increase their odds of surviving long enough to get fat enough for market. With these antibiotics in such widespread use, there is massive opportunity for resistant strains to emerge and flourish.

We call them superbugs. And we humans are increasingly vulnerable to their antibiotic-resistant ways. Farm animals are also pumped full of antiviral drugs, leading to the emergence of drug-resistant strains of viruses. Combined with the stress of confinement impairing the animals' immune systems, these farms are perfect incubators for new viruses, which are now mutating like never before and becoming increasingly difficult to control.

I'm no expert on viruses and bacteria, so for this chapter I rely particularly heavily on an interview with someone who is—Michael Greger, MD. I recently read Dr. Greger's book *Bird Flu: A Virus of Our Own Hatching* (it can be found free online at www.birdflubook.org), which is about the potential of a deadly flu pandemic, the likes of which we have never seen, and I went directly to him to find out more. In the book, Dr. Greger very clearly delineates how a new virus begins, mutates, and becomes dangerous. And as with so many problems we are seeing lately—water pollution, climate change, you name it—factory-farmed meat seems to be a big part of the cause.

A graduate of the Cornell University School of Agriculture and the Tufts University School of Medicine, Michael Greger serves as the director of public health and animal agriculture at the Humane Society of the United States. His recent articles in the *American Journal of Preventive Medicine*, *Biosecurity and Bioterrorism*, *Critical Reviews in Microbiology*, and *the International Journal of Food Safety, Nutrition, and Public Health* explore the public health implications of industrialized animal agriculture.

According to Dr. Greger, more than 95 percent of the meat, dairy, and eggs we eat comes from factory farms. Not only are dangerous flu viruses mutating because of these concentrated animal feeding operations (CAFOs) but we are also being exposed to some other very serious bacteria and pathogens. The good news is that by eating a plant-based diet, we significantly reduce our risk of exposure and vote with our dollars against a business model that is causing such health havoc.

Straight from the Source: Michael Greger, MD, on Factory Farming and Superbugs

Here's what Dr. Greger says about the bugs that are germinating now.

KF: How likely are we to have a bird or swine flu that turns into something really deadly and widespread?
MG: Unfortunately we don't know enough about the biology of these viruses to make accurate predictions, but influenza is definitely the disease to keep an eye on. AIDS has killed millions but is only fluid borne. Malaria has killed millions but is relatively restricted to equatorial regions. Flu viruses are the only known pathogen capable of infecting literally billions of people in a matter of months. Right now [early 2010] we are in the midst of a flu pandemic caused by the swine-origin influenza virus H1N1. Tens of millions of people have become infected and thousands of young people have died, but H1N1 is not particularly virulent. There are other flu viruses that have emerged in recent decades such as the highly "pathogenic" (disease-causing) bird flu H5N1 that may have the potential to cause much greater human harm.

KF: What kind of damage could it do in terms of population mortality?

MG: Currently H5N1 kills approximately 60 percent of those it infects, so you don't even get a coin toss chance of survival. That's a mortality rate on par with some strains of Ebola. Fortunately, only a few hundred people have become infected. Should a virus like H5N1 trigger a pandemic, though, the results could be catastrophic.

During a pandemic as many as 2 or 3 billion people can become infected. A 60 percent mortality rate is simply unimaginable. Unfortunately, it's not as far-fetched as it sounds. Both China and Indonesia have reported sporadic outbreaks of the H5N1 bird flu in pigs and sporadic outbreaks of the new pandemic virus H1N1 in pigs as well. Theoretically, if a pig became coinfected with both strains, a hybrid mutant could arise with the human transmissibility of swine flu and the human lethality of bird flu. That's the kind of nightmare scenario that keeps virologists up at night.

KF: How does a virus like that kill? What does it do to the body?

MG: Most often it starts with standard flulike symptoms—fever, cough, and muscle aches. Instead of just infecting the respiratory tract, though, H5N1 may spread throughout the body and infect the brain, for example, leaving victims in a coma. Other early symptoms atypical of regular seasonal flu include vomiting, diarrhea, abdominal pain, chest pain, and bleeding from the nose and gums. Death is usually from acute fulminant respiratory distress, in which one basically drowns in one's own blood-tinted respiratory secretions.

Most of the damage is actually done by one's own immune system. H5N1 seems to trigger a "cytokine storm," an overexuberant immune reaction to the virus. These cytokine chemical messengers set off such a massive inflammatory reaction that on autopsy the lungs of victims may be virus-free, meaning that your body wins, but in burning down the village in order to save it you may not live through the process. Indeed, the reason why young people may be so vulnerable is because they have the strongest immune systems, and it's your immune system that may kill you.

KF: How easy is it to contract the virus?
MG: Catching a pandemic flu virus is essentially as easy as catching the regular seasonal flu. During a flu pandemic about one in five people may fall ill, but there are certainly ways to minimize your risk, by washing your hands and social distancing techniques. In a really severe pandemic, though, the advice would be to "shelter-in-place," isolating yourself and your family in your home until the danger passes. During such a pandemic the Department of Homeland Security uses as a key planning assumption that the American population would be asked to self-quarantine for up to ninety days per wave of the pandemic.

KF: Why do we have this potential disaster on our hands?
MG: The industrialization of the chicken and pork industries is thought to have wrought these unprecedented

changes in avian and swine influenza. No one even got sick from bird flu for eight decades before a new strain H5N1 started killing children in 1997. Likewise, in pigs here in the U.S., swine flu was totally stable for eight decades before a pig-bird-human hybrid mutant virus appeared in commercial pig populations in 1998. It was that strain that combined with a Eurasian swine flu virus ten years later to spawn the flu pandemic of 2009, which sickened millions of young people around the world.

The first hybrid mutant swine flu virus discovered in the United States was at a factory farm in North Carolina in which thousands of pregnant sows were confined in "gestation crates," veal-crate-like metal stalls barely larger than their bodies. These kind of stressful, filthy, overcrowded conditions can provide a breeding ground for the emergence and spread of new diseases.

So far, only thousands of people have died from swine flu. Unless we radically change the way chickens and pigs are raised for food, though, it may only be a matter of time before a catastrophic pandemic arises.

KF: If factory farms are to blame, why have there been plagues and flus throughout time, when factory farms were not around?
MG: Before the domestication of birds, about 2,500 years ago, human influenza likely didn't even exist. Similarly, before the domestication of livestock there were no measles, smallpox, or many other diseases that have plagued humanity since they were born in the barnyard about 10,000 years ago. Once dis-

eases jump the species barrier from the animal kingdom, they can spread independently throughout human populations with tragic consequences.

The worst plague in human history was the 1918 flu pandemic triggered by a bird flu virus that went on to kill upwards of 50 million people. The crowded, stressful, unhygienic trench warfare conditions during World War I that led to the emergence of the 1918 virus are replicated today in nearly every industrial chicken shed and egg operation. Instead of millions of vulnerable hosts to evolve within back then, we now have *billions* of chickens intensively confined in factory farms, arguably the perfect-storm environment for the emergence and spread of hypervirulent, so-called predator-type viruses like H5N1. The 1918 virus killed about 2.5 percent of the people it infected, twenty times deadlier than the seasonal flu. H5N1 is now killing 60 percent of infected people, twenty times deadlier than the 1918 virus. So if a virus like 1918's gained easy human transmissibility, it could make the 1918 pandemic—the deadliest plague ever—look like the regular flu.

KF: Does handling or eating chicken or pork increase a person's chances of contracting the virus?
MG: There are certainly lots of viruses people can pick up from handling fresh meat, such as those that cause unpleasant conditions like contagious pustular dermatitis and a well-defined medical condition known as "butcher's warts." Even the wives of butchers appear to be at higher risk for cervical cancer, a cancer definitively associated with wart virus exposure.

Cooking can destroy the flu virus, and the same can be said for all the other bugs that sicken 76 million Americans a year. The problem is that people can cross-contaminate kitchen surfaces with fresh or frozen meat before pathogens have been cooked to death. There have been a number of cases of human influenza linked to the consumption of poultry products, but swine flu viruses don't appear to get into the meat. Regardless, the primary risk is not in the meat, but how meat is produced. Once a new disease is spawned from factory farm conditions it may be able to spread person to person, and at that point animals—live or dead—may be out of the picture.

KF: How do we stave off the risk?
MG: We need to give these animals more breathing room. The Pew Commission on Industrial Farm Animal Production, which included a former U.S. secretary of agriculture, concluded that industrialized animal agriculture posed "unacceptable" public health risks, and called for gestation crates for pigs to be banned as they're already doing in Europe, noting that "[p]ractices that restrict natural motion, such as sow gestation crates, induce high levels of stress in the animals and threaten their health, which in turn may threaten human health."

Studies have shown that measures as simple as providing straw for pigs so they don't have the immune-crippling stress of living on bare concrete their whole lives can significantly cut down on swine flu transmission rates. Such a minimal act—providing straw—yet we often deny these animals even this modicum of mercy, both to their detriment and, potentially, to ours as well.

The American Public Health Association, the largest organization of public health professionals in the world, has called for a moratorium on factory farms. In fact the APHA journal, the *American Journal of Public Health*, published an editorial that not only called for an end to factory farms, it questioned the prudence of raising so many animals in the first place:

> It is curious . . . that changing the way humans treat animals—most basically, ceasing to eat them or, at the very least, radically limiting the quantity of them that are eaten—is largely off the radar as a significant preventive measure. Such a change, if sufficiently adopted or imposed, could still reduce the chances of the much-feared influenza epidemic. It would be even more likely to prevent unknown future diseases that, in the absence of this change, may result from farming animals intensively and from killing them for food. Yet humanity does not consider this option. . . . Those who consume animals not only harm those animals and endanger themselves, but they also threaten the well-being of other humans who currently or will later inhabit the planet. . . . [I]t is time for humans to remove their heads from the sand and recognize the risk to themselves that can arise from their maltreatment of other species.

KF: That is a pretty stunning statement! I know people will wonder "If we give up animal protein, will our immune systems be compromised . . . or enhanced?"

MG: We've known for twenty years that the immune function of those eating vegetarian may be superior to those eating meat. In a study first published in 1989, researchers at the German Cancer Research Center found that although vegetarians had the same number of disease-fighting white blood cells as meat eaters, the immune cells of vegetarians were twice as effective in destroying their targets—not only cancer cells, but virus-infected cells as well. So a more plant-based diet may protect both now and in the future against animal-borne diseases like pandemic influenza.

KF: Where does *E. coli* come from and how does it get into food? Why is it often found on vegetables?

In a study published in 1989, researchers at the German Cancer Research Center found that although vegetarians had the same number of disease-fighting white blood cells as meat eaters, the immune cells of vegetarians were twice as effective in destroying their targets— not only cancer cells, but virus-infected cells as well.

MG: *E. coli* is an intestinal pathogen. It only gets in the food if fecal matter gets in the food. Since plants don't have intestines, all *E. coli* infections—in fact all food poisoning—comes from animals. When's the last time you heard of anyone getting Dutch elm disease or a really bad case of aphids? People don't get plant diseases; they get animal diseases. The problem is that because of the number of animals raised today, a billion tons of manure is produced every year in the United States—the weight of 10,000 Nimitz-class aircraft carriers. Dairy cow and pig factories often dump millions of gallons of putrefying waste into massive open-air cesspits, which can leak and contaminate water used to irrigate our crops. That's how a deadly fecal pathogen like *E. coli* O157:H7 can end up contaminating our spinach. So regardless of what we eat, we all need to fight against the expansion of factory farming in our communities, our nation, and around the world.

KF: What percentage of the population gets hit by the bacteria? How many of them die? Could that likely increase?

MG: While *E. coli* O157:H7 remains the leading cause of acute kidney failure in U.S. children, fewer than 100,000 Americans get infected every year, and fewer than 100 die. But millions get infected with other types of *E. coli* that can cause urinary tract infections (UTIs) that can invade the bloodstream and cause an estimated 36,000 deaths annually in the United States.

KF: It seems we only occasionally hear of the very few terrible cases where *E. coli* kills; is it really a widespread problem?

MG: When medical researchers at the University of Minnesota took more than 1,000 food samples from multiple retail markets, they found evidence of fecal contamination in 69 percent of the pork and beef and 92 percent of the poultry samples. Nine out of ten chicken carcasses in the store may be contaminated with fecal matter. And half of the poultry samples were contaminated with the UTI-causing *E. coli* bacteria.

Scientists now suspect that by eating chicken, women infect their lower intestinal tract with these meat-borne bacteria, which can then creep up into their bladder. Hygiene measures to prevent UTIs have traditionally included wiping from front to back after bowel movements and urinating after intercourse to flush out any invaders, but now women can add poultry avoidance as a way to help prevent urinary tract infections.

KF: Are there any long-term problems for people who ingest *E. coli* and have a bad day or two with diarrhea, or is the problem over once *E. coli* is out of the system?
MG: Recently the Center for Foodborne Illness Research and Prevention released a report on the long-term consequences of common causes of food poisoning. Lifelong complications of *E. coli* O157:H7 infection include end-stage kidney disease, permanent brain damage, and insulin-dependent diabetes.

KF: Is *E. coli* a problem if the meat is cooked?
MG: With the exception of prions, the infectious agents responsible for mad cow disease and the human equivalent—which can survive even incineration at temperatures hot enough to melt lead—all viral, fungal, and bacterial pathogens in our food supply can be killed by proper cooking. Why then do tens of millions of Americans come down with food poisoning every year? Cross-contamination is thought to account for the bulk of infections. For example, chicken carcasses

are so covered in bacteria that researchers at the University of Arizona found more fecal bacteria in the kitchen—on sponges and dish towels, and in the sink drain—than they found swabbing the toilet. In a meat eater's house it may be safer to lick the rim of the toilet seat than the kitchen countertop, because people aren't preparing chickens in their toilets. Chicken "juice" is essentially raw fecal soup.

KF: What goes on inside the body when a human ingests *E. coli*?
[Note to reader: You might not want to read this next section on a full stomach. It's very graphic and deeply disturbing.]
MG: Depending on the strain, the number of bacteria ingested, and the immune status of the victim, it can fail to cause any disease at all or, in the worst cases, cause multisystem organ failure. Here's how one mother described what *E. coli* O157:H7 did to her three-year-old daughter Brianna: "The pain during the first eighty hours was horrific, with intense abdominal cramping every ten to twelve minutes. Her intestines swelled to three times their normal size and she was placed on a ventilator. Emergency surgery became essential and her colon was removed. After further surgery, doctors decided to leave the incision open, from sternum to pubis, to allow Brianna's swollen organs room to expand and prevent them from ripping her skin. Her heart was so swollen it was like a sponge and bled from every pore. Her liver and pancreas shut down and she was gripped by thousands of convulsions, which caused blood clots in her eyes. We were told she was brain dead."

KF: What a horror. Why is it deadly for some and not others?

MG: We think it has to do with the virulence of the bacteria—some strains are deadlier than others—and the vulnerability of the host. We're not sure why children under five years of age are at the highest risk for dangerous complications, but that is certainly a finding that has been consistent.

KF: Is factory-farmed meat more likely to get _E. coli_ out into the market, or is all meat (even free-range) carrying that potential?

MG: In chickens, these bacteria cause a disease called colibacillosis, now one of the most significant and widespread infectious diseases in the poultry industry because of the way we now raise these animals. Studies have shown infection risk to be directly linked to overcrowding on factory chicken farms. In caged egg-laying hens, the most significant risk factor for flock infection is hen density per cage. Researchers have calculated that affording just a single quart of additional living space to each hen would be associated with a corresponding 33 percent drop in the risk of colibacillosis outbreak. This is one of the reasons many efforts to improve the lives of farmed animals is critical not only for animal welfare, but for the health of humans and animals alike.

In terms of other infections, such as campylobacter, the most common cause of bacterial food poisoning in the United States, _Consumer Reports_ published an analysis of retail chicken in their January 2010 issue. They found that the majority of store-bought chickens were contaminated with campylobacter, which can trigger arthritis, heart and blood infections, and a condition called Guillain-Barré syndrome, which can leave people permanently disabled and paralyzed. Comparing store brands, [they found that] 59 percent of the conventional factory-farmed chickens were contaminated, compared with 57 percent of chickens raised organically. So there might be a marginal difference, but the best strategy may be to avoid meat completely. With the virtual elimination of polio, the most common cause of neuromuscular paralysis in the United States now comes from eating chicken.

KF: **What about salmonella? Is it really a big deal, or is it just a matter of an upset stomach?**
MG: Salmonella kills more Americans than any other foodborne illness. There is an epidemic of egg-borne food poisoning every year in the United States. To this day, more than 100,000 Americans per year are sickened annually by salmonella-infected eggs.

KF: **Do we have more salmonella now than we did twenty-five or fifty years ago? If so, why?**

"Salmonella kills more Americans than any other foodborne illness. There is an epidemic of egg-borne food poisoning every year in the United States. To this day, more than 100,000 Americans are sickened annually by salmonella-infected eggs."—Michael Greger, MD

MG: There was a time when our grandparents could drink eggnog and children could eat raw cookie dough without fear of joining the thousands of Americans hospitalized with salmonella infections every year. Before the industrialization of egg production, salmonella only sickened a few hundred Americans every year and *Salmonella enteritidis* was not found in eggs at all. By the beginning of the twenty-first century, however, *Salmonella enteritidis*–contaminated eggs were sickening an estimated 182,000 Americans annually.

There are many industrial practices that contribute to the alarming rates of this disease. Most eggs come from hens confined in battery cages, small barren wire enclosures affording these animals less living space than a single sheet of letter-size paper for virtually their entire one- to two-year life span. Salmonella-contaminated battery cage operations in the United States confine an average of more than 100,000 hens in a single shed. The massive volume of contaminated airborne fecal dust in such a facility rapidly accelerates the spread of infection.

Factory-farming practices also led to the spread of salmonella around the world. Just as the feeding of dead animals to live ones triggered the mad cow crisis, this same practice has also been implicated in the global spread of salmonella. Once egg production wanes, hens may be ground up and rendered into what is called "spent hen meal," and then fed to other hens. More than half of the feed samples for farmed birds containing slaughter-plant waste tested by the FDA were found to be contaminated with salmonella. CDC researchers have estimated that more than 1,000,000 cases of salmonella poisoning in Americans can be directly tied to feed containing animal by-products.

KF: What happens to the body when salmonella gets into the system?
MG: Within twelve to seventy-two hours of infection the fever, diarrhea, and abdominal cramps start. If the victim is lucky it's over within a week. If not, the bacteria can burrow through the intestinal wall and infect the bloodstream, seeding its way to other organs, including the heart, bones, and brain.

KF: Are there any long-term consequences from exposure?
MG: Thanks to salmonella infection, one breakfast omelet can now trigger persistent irritable bowel syndrome and what's called reactive arthritis, which can become a debilitating lifelong condition of swollen painful joints. Because salmonella can infect the ovaries of hens, eggs from infected birds can be laid prepackaged with the bacteria inside. According to research funded by the American Egg Board, salmonella can survive sunny-side up, over-easy, and scrambled egg cooking methods.

KF: Would free-range meat or eggs be less likely to be contaminated?
MG: There is evidence that eggs from cage-free hens pose less of a threat. In the largest study of its kind (analyzing more than 30,000 samples taken from more than 5,000 operations across two dozen countries in Europe) cage-free barns had

about 40 percent lower odds of harboring the egg-related strain of salmonella.

KF: Can we get salmonella just from touching something tainted?
MG: Absolutely; in fact the infective dose for salmonella is as few as fifteen to twenty bacteria, and a single egg can be infected with hundreds. It's important to understand where the egg comes out. Eggs emerge from the hen's vent, which is kind of a joint opening for both her vagina and anus, which explains the level of fecal contamination one can find on eggs.

CDC researchers have estimated that more than 1 million cases of salmonella poisoning in Americans can be directly tied to feed containing animal by-products.

KF: Is it contagious?
MG: Person-to-person transmission of salmonella can occur when an infected person's feces, unwashed from his or her hands, contaminates food during preparation or comes into direct contact with another person.

KF: Who is most at risk for serious illness or even death?
MG: More than half of all reported salmonella infections occur in children, who are especially susceptible to serious complications. Elderly and immunocompromised adults are

also particularly vulnerable. In the United States, though, some strains of salmonella are growing dangerously resistant to up to six major classes of antibiotics, due in large part to the irresponsible factory-farming practice of feeding millions of pounds of antibiotics to animals every year as a crutch to combat the stressful and overcrowded conditions of intensive animal agriculture systems. This puts everyone at risk.

KF: What is the overall solution to prevent these dangerous pathogens and bacteria?
MG: Over the last few decades new animal-to-human infectious diseases have emerged at an unprecedented rate. According to the World Health Organization, the increasing global demand for animal protein is a key underlying factor.

Swine flu is not the only deadly human disease traced to factory-farming practices. The meat industry took natural herbivores like cows and sheep and turned them into carnivores and cannibals by feeding them slaughterhouse waste, blood, and manure. Then they fed people "downer" animals—too sick to even walk. Now the world has mad cow disease.

In 2005 the world's largest and deadliest outbreak of a pathogen called *Streptococcus suis* emerged, causing meningitis and deafness in people handling infected pork products. Experts blamed the emergence on factory-farming practices. Pig factories in Malaysia birthed the Nipah virus, one of the deadliest of human pathogens, a contagious respiratory disease that causes relapsing brain infections and kills 40 percent of people infected. Its emergence was likewise blamed squarely on factory farming.

The pork industry in the U.S. feeds pigs millions of pounds

of human antibiotics every year just to promote growth in such a stressful, unhygienic environment, and now there are these multi-drug-resistant bacteria and we as physicians are running out of good antibiotic options. As the UK's chief medical officer put it in his 2009 annual report: "Every inappropriate use of antibiotics in agriculture is a potential death warrant for a future patient."

In the short term we need to put an end to the riskiest practices, such as extreme confinement—gestation crates and battery cages—and the nontherapeutic feeding of antibiotics. We have to follow the advice of the American Public Health Association to declare a moratorium on factory farms and eventually phase them out completely.

This was just mind-blowing to me, to hear how dangerous viruses are growing in meat and egg production facilities, and to know that animals are so dosed with antibiotics that resistant strains of bacteria are becoming out of control. It almost sounds like science fiction. Another excellent reason to shift toward a plant-based diet.

PROMISE 5:

You Will Save Money

Did you know?

- You can satisfy your protein needs with an enormous variety of delicious vegetarian foods for just pennies per day.
- The annual costs of meat-based diseases in the U.S., direct and indirect, are on the order of $1 trillion, and climbing—costs that show up in the exorbitant price of health care. We can only hope that when we cut out meat and dairy, by decreasing the amount of disease, we will eventually see lower medical bills.
- According to the former World Bank economist Raj Patel, that "cheap" burger that costs you a few bucks at a restaurant actually costs over $200 to bring to your plate when all true resource costs are accounted for. Eating vegan also lightens your overall environmental debt.

As I talk to people about becoming a veganist, one common refrain I hear is that it's too expensive. When funds are low, the cheap burger or basket of chicken can appear to be the best value—the greatest density of filling calories for the lowest price. We've been aggressively peddled the idea that a healthy diet is an expensive diet, something only for rich folks. And our experience seems to bear that out.

I understand the frustration. It doesn't seem right that meat should be so cheap (it's not, but more on that later) and fresh vegetables, especially organic ones, relatively expensive. But once you look into it, the true cost of eating animal protein is higher than you can imagine. And being veganist in your approach to food is not only healthier by every measure but it can be considerably cheaper as well. In fact, many staples of a vegan diet cost very little and can be found in any grocery store—not just in specialty markets. Whole grains like quinoa or barley or brown rice, legumes like chickpeas or soybeans, and other beans like black-eyed peas and black beans are very inexpensive—certainly cheaper than processed and packaged foods. Bought in bulk, whole grains and beans can cost just pennies per meal. And because they are full of fiber, they make you feel full and satisfied (put them into soups, stews, salads, burritos, etc.), without the dangerous saturated fat of animal protein. Fresh vegetables and fruits can be found at supermarkets and farmers' markets for very reasonable prices (see money-saving tips at the end of this chapter). Organic and specialty stores are great, but it's certainly not necessary to empty your wallet in order to eat healthy.

In the mid-1990s, *Vegetarian Times* magazine set out to

determine the cost of being a vegetarian. Two friends—one vegetarian and one not—agreed to go shopping for a week's worth of groceries to feed their respective families of four. They shopped at the same store and made similar purchases, although the vegetarian bought soy sausages and black beans instead of chicken cutlets and ground turkey. The bottom line was that the vegetarian spent 17 percent percent less than her meat-eating friend did, and most of that difference was due to the price of meat. When extrapolated out over an entire year, they estimated that the vegetarian family saved about $1,180 (in mid-1990s dollars) on their annual food bill.

Beans, grains, veggies—these are the staples of populations around the world. Think of Mexico and South America, where inexpensive rice and beans coupled with corn tortillas and avocados are part of every diet; or rural China, where tofu with vegetables and rice, and maybe a very small bit of meat, is the norm; or India where people eat dal (lentils) with rice and vegetables every day. Not only are these populations by no means uniformly wealthy, they don't have the diseases of wealthy countries. The general populations who eat these simple diets may get waterborne illnesses and lung infections from bad environmental conditions, but they don't have anywhere near the rates of cancer, heart disease, and diabetes that we have—until they are exposed to our Western diet, that is.

And that's something to think about. Not only is a healthful plant-based diet less expensive at the grocery store (unless you go crazy for packaged convenience foods, of course), it saves you personally and saves us societally in health care and many other direct and indirect costs. If you think these don't affect you so much, think again. On the individual level alone, consider that your health insurance never pays for everything: even the best of plans charge deductibles and disallow certain medications. Being sick is expensive. More than that, a huge part of our country's annual budget is given over to health-care costs, paid for by your tax dollars. And indirect health-care costs due to lost productivity adversely affect you in the form of higher taxes, too.

On the health-care front, when you consider that meat and dairy foods clog our bodies with saturated fat, growth hormones, and antibiotics, things that have been conclusively linked to cancer, heart disease, and obesity, as well as a general "blah" feeling, it's certainly a lot less expensive—and less painful—to *prevent* debilitating diseases through our food choices than it is to treat them later (through bypass surgery or angioplasty, for example, which can run up tens of thousands of dollars in medical bills).

Remember in the last chapter where we looked at the link between diet and Alzheimer's? Well Alzheimer's doesn't just steal one's memory or personality (as if that weren't enough), it also costs more than you can imagine. According to a report by the Alzheimer's Association, "from 2010 to 2050, the cost of caring for Americans sixty-five and older with Alzheimer's disease will increase more than six times, to $1.08 trillion. Currently, $172 billion a year is spent by the government, private insurance and individuals to care for people with the disease, the most common cause of dementia."

What about other health conditions?

A 2010 study from Emory University in Atlanta shows that obesity-related health-care costs in the U.S. have hit $145 billion and are expected to top $340 billion by 2018. That will represent more than one-fifth of all health-care spending annually, and about half of it will be publicly financed. Indirect costs from lost productivity attributable to obesity will roughly double that figure.

Heart disease costs more than $500 billion annually, and the disease is almost totally preventable with a plant-based diet. And cancer? More than $225 billion. Diabetes? About $175 billion, with an indisputable link to diet.

Disease is expensive, both to the individuals and families dealing with it and to agencies like Medicare and Medicaid, which are ultimately funded by us, the taxpayers. When you look at the skyrocketing costs of treating heart disease, cancer, diabetes, as well as diseases like Alzheimer's, it's clear that it makes far more sense, both morally and monetarily, on both a personal and societal level, to take preventive measures such as changing the way we eat.

It just makes sense to factor in the true costs of a meat-based diet.

In the long term, it's a lot less expensive—and less painful—to *prevent* debilitating diseases through our food choices than it is to treat them later.

In short, at the very least, a fat- and calorie-filled meat-based diet makes us feel bad. It lowers our energy and keeps us from thriving, both physically and financially. A plant-based

The domino effect of government subsidies to grain farmers to meat [crossed out] farmers + fish farmers

diet, on the other hand, gives us a feeling of lightness, clear-headedness, and energy. Over time, meat-based diets can cost us our health, whereas a vegan diet delivers healthy longevity.

Why *Is* Meat So Cheap?

Getting back to the wallet, why *is* meat so cheap?

Because it's subsidized.

That's right. Not only does the meat industry get away with not paying the full costs of its operations—costs to animal welfare, to our health, to the watershed, to the land—it also benefits from a steady blizzard of government subsidies.

Wait! Don't turn the page.

If you're like me, your eyes probably glaze over at a word like *subsidies.* But subsidies are actually pretty interesting business—and not at all hard to understand.

A government subsidy is a form of financial assistance paid to an industry to help prevent that industry's decline. The U.S. government provides all kinds of subsidies—to cover housing, water, etc.—using taxpayer money. When it comes to agricultural subsidies, our tax dollars literally keep the meat industry afloat.

Here's how it works: With help from government subsidies, many farmers are able to sell their corn and soybeans for far less than the cost of production. The subsidies—paid for with our tax dollars—compensate them for the difference. As a result of these artificially cheap prices, owners of factory farms are able to then purchase at bargain-basement prices the grain they need to feed their chickens, turkeys, pigs, and cows. This gives them an enormous advantage over

50 % of fish today comes from farms

foreign competitors (not to mention a huge leg up over small organic ranchers who wouldn't think of feeding conventional [often genetically modified] feed to their animals, but that's another story).

One lucky recipient of such subsidies is Tyson Foods, the world's largest poultry company. Like many other meat companies, Tyson has collected billions of dollars worth of government subsidies in the last decade alone. Why does Tyson get such heavy subsidies, but companies that make healthy plant-based foods don't? It seems so wrong. And yet from 1997 through 2005, Tyson Foods effectively collected government subsidies worth $2.59 billion.

Subsidies have given these industries such a boost that others naturally want to get in on the action. Half the fish consumed worldwide now comes from fish farms, which are lining up for their share of government subsidies. And government officials want to expand the U.S. aquaculture industry to five times its current size. It seems we have to get ready to open our wallets yet again.

These fish farms are already beneficiaries of government aid. The U.S. Department of Agriculture's Small Business Innovation Research program has given away millions of dollars in grants to fish-farming companies. Even the much-maligned "stimulus" (officially, the American Recovery and Reinvestment Act of 2009) set aside $50 million for states to help compensate fish farmers for losses associated with the high cost of feed. These are forms of subsidies as well.

It seems that eating fish is not only a health and environmental hazard (PCBs, mercury, destruction of the aquatic food chain, antibiotics and other medicines necessary to aquaculture, etc.), but a fiscal hazard as well.

Okay, you say, so these industries get a little help. What's so bad about that? For starters, that same public assistance is not available to fruit and vegetable growers! If it were, consumers—especially those in impoverished communities—wouldn't feel that they had to choose between "cheap" burgers or "healthy" and "humane" fruits and veggies at the checkout line.

In other words, the prices are rigged, and those of us who want to eat the most healthy diet possible sometimes have to pay the price. That's why it's so important that we vote with our dollars.

Every time we go to the grocery store or out to eat, we get a chance to vote against wasteful spending, simply by not buying meat, eggs, and dairy products.

We may not be able to direct large-scale government spending anytime soon, but one area where we do have control is in how we spend at the market. Every time we go to the grocery store or out to eat, we get a chance to vote against wasteful spending, simply by not buying meat, eggs, and dairy products. Eventually, these individual acts of ours *will* change the economics of agriculture, with vegetables and fruits and nuts and grains competing on a level playing field against animal agriculture.

The High Price of Poop

The government's gross spending only gets grosser when we're faced with this scary statistic: pound for pound, a pig produces four times as much waste as a person does. According to the Union of Concerned Scientists, factory farms generate about 300 million tons of manure every year. That's more than double the amount produced by the country's entire human population!

Plus, densely stocked fish farms—the fastest growing form of agriculture in the world—also produce tremendous amounts of waste—everything from uneaten, chemical-laden fish feed to fish feces—that can wreak havoc on local ecosystems.

What does that have to do with you and me? All the waste produced on these farms has to go somewhere. And guess who pays for the cleanup? It's not the factory farmers . . .

Highly polluting factory farms are being prioritized for government funding, but no federal guidelines regulate how factory farms spend that money to treat, store, and dispose of the one trillion pounds of animal excrement that they produce every year. Factory farms often pump animal waste into huge, putrid manure lagoons, or spray it over crops as fertilizer. Both of these disposal methods result in run-off that contaminates the soil and water and kills fish and other wildlife. There are numerous reports that humans who live near factory farms have become sick from the pollution—many suffer from respiratory ailments, neurological problems, and as suggested by a 2010 review in the *Journal of Animal Science*, the stench from these factory farms can cause sexual dysfunction: "Some odors may destroy normal positive pheromone responses resulting

Americans on average eat over 200 pounds of meat per year.

in impaired sexual function for people living in the vicinity of CAFO." More hidden costs.

Americans eat, on average, some 200 pounds of meat, poultry, and fish (not to mention eggs and dairy products) per person per year. Part of the reason for this high consumption of animal protein is, of course, the low cost.

Corporate welfare in the form of agricultural subsidies, as well as cost-cutting practices on factory farms that include crowding animals together by the thousands in filthy warehouses and grinding up the scraps from dead animals and feeding them back to the survivors, have made meat cheap and readily available. What all this means is that the true and unacceptably high "cost" of meat—to our health, to the welfare of animals, to our precious ecosystem— is hidden behind a wall of price manipulations and other illusions. And even so, it can be cheaper not to eat meat at all.

Money-Saving Tips

Making the switch to a plant-based diet might seem challenging at first, but it's actually so simple, and a few smart shopping strategies can also help you save on food bills.

1. **Buy in season. Produce in season is almost always** less expensive than out-of-season produce, **because it's more abundant.**
2. **Avoid precut, washed, and packaged fruits and vegetables. They're always more expensive than the whole foods (and a waste of packaging). If you need the convenience (for the office, or if you're**

on the road), go for it; just know that you'll be
paying more.

3. Watch produce prices carefully. Locally grown
   fruits and vegetables sometimes cost less than
   imported produce, while at other times imported
   produce saves you a lot—just be on the lookout
   for the best deals. (And be mindful of the carbon
   footprint—how far your food had to travel to you
   and therefore how much fuel was required to get
   it there.)

4. Shop at farmers' markets at the end of the day.
   Farmers' markets are a great place to find fresh,
   in-season, and locally grown produce for cheap—
   especially if you shop at the end of the market
   day, when growers may be willing to sell their
   produce at a discount, rather than have to pack
   it up and take it back home with them.

5. Don't be afraid to buy frozen vegetables. Frozen
   veggies (especially store brands) are often cheaper
   than fresh ones, and they can actually be *more*
   nutritious, because the veggies are frozen right after they're picked, preserving vitamins that are
   lost in transporting fresh veggies from the farm to
   the store. And of course, keep an eye out for sales
   and stock up your freezer with veggies that can
   be tossed into soups, stews, stir-fries, pasta, and
   many other dishes.

6. Consider the value of your time. For most of us,
   time is just as valuable as money. We tend to think
   that eating fast food is less time-consuming—an

illusion reinforced by a steady stream of fast-food company advertising. But in reality, the time that you spend driving to a fast-food restaurant and then idling in a drive-through could just as easily be spent at home with your family, cooking a simple meal. All it takes is a small initial time investment in learning to cook a few new meals. Even simpler, you can just convert the meals that you already eat into ones that fit your new lifestyle.

Most families rotate the same menu of dishes every week, for ease of preparation and to simplify grocery shopping. Once you've got that set menu of favorite vegan meals, prep time is quick.

7. Veganize the meals you already eat. When my friends Robbie and Colleen made the decision to eat vegan meals, they worried about how they'd feed their family while remaining in their budget. One of the first things that Robbie and Colleen did was to consider how they could take the meat and dairy out of the meals that they already served without spending any extra money.

For example, tacos with ground beef became tacos with seasoned black beans, which worked out to be less expensive, even when they used canned beans, and far healthier than using a package of ground beef. Instead of sour cream and cheese, Robbie and Colleen made a delicious substitution of homemade guacamole—this before they discovered vegan versions of sour cream and cheese. To replace their usual chicken breasts at dinner, they substituted grilled tofu or seitan "steaks," which are cheaper than a package of boneless chicken breasts. Their kids loved the seitan (made from the protein in wheat) especially, and it quickly became part of the regular rotation.

Spaghetti and meatballs, a longtime favorite of the whole family, became spaghetti with meatless marinara sauce, made either with fresh tomatoes (which can be bought inexpensively at many farmers' markets) or a delicious sauce made with diced, canned tomatoes (often on sale in their local supermarket) mixed up with crumbled tofu; when the tofu was mixed in, it seemed like the classic Bolognese sauce. Sometimes they used vegetarian meatballs instead, and it was as hearty and delicious as anything they'd had before.

Again, removing the meat from the meal made it no more expensive than if they'd added the fatty, unhealthy meat—with its attendant costly, long-term health problems. For those occasions when they would be pressed for time, Robbie and Colleen took to the Internet to look for some quick, on-the-go vegan options. They found that the nutritional information for every fast-food restaurant was online, and just a few clicks uncovered quite a few vegan fast-food options. The chain Chipotle, with its vegan-friendly menu and have-it-your-way meal options, was always a reliable, inexpensive place to eat. It was even possible to have vegan meals at "standard" chain restaurants—Denny's has a veggie burger, for instance; and veggie fast-food restaurants seemed to be coming onto the scene, many of them squeezed into strip shopping malls or other convenient places. Often Colleen would just make a huge pot of chili that would last for the week; or Robbie would barbecue skewers of veggies and tempeh on the grill in nearly no time. They made chopped salads or fresh veggies every day to fill out the menus.

8. Think quantity. Nonperishable foods like dried beans, rice, and oatmeal are far cheaper if bought in bulk. If you plan your weekly meals in advance and make a list of what you'll need—and stick to it when you go shopping to avoid pricey splurges or food that you won't use up before it spoils—you'll save quite a bit of money. Dried beans and lentils, for example, cost less than $1 a pound, and they are a great source of protein. Tofu—the "other white meat" of the vegan universe and one of those blank-slate foods, like flour, to which you add flavors to make interesting—usually costs less than $2 a pound. If you are fortunate enough to live near a Chinatown, you can sometimes find super fresh, locally made tofu for less than $1 a pound. If you live near a Trader Joe's, you can find great deals on healthy,

vegetarian foods—and you'll probably discover some new favorites that your regular grocery store doesn't carry.

9. Invest in some good vegan cookbooks (my favorites are listed at the back of this book, and there are many week's worth of recipes in the back of both my *Quantum Wellness* books) so that you'll be more likely to make meals at home instead of going out to eat or buying expensive convenience foods. There are also great websites that offer recipes for free, and I've listed them at the back of this book as well.

Of course, many inexpensive, healthy, and easy-to-make meals don't even require a recipe. For breakfast, try toast or a bagel spread with vegan butter, peanut butter, jam, or avocado, or have a bowl of cereal topped with sliced bananas. My regular breakfast is cold brown rice (I make enough for a week at a time and keep it in the refrigerator) with chopped dates, raw almonds, and hemp or rice milk (I heat up the milk). A baked potato topped with salsa, baked beans, or vegan chili makes a tasty and filling lunch or dinner along with a salad; tacos loaded with beans, rice, and veggies are inexpensive and delicious. Good old peanut butter and jelly sandwiches or cheesy toast made with soy or tapioca cheeses are a hit with kids of all ages and are easy on the wallet.

Once you find your basics that you can depend on in a pinch, you will find that you can even splurge on some specialty products, such as veggie burgers and mock chicken,

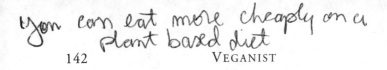
you can eat more cheaply on a plant based diet

and still spend less than you would if you loaded up on beef, chicken, and fish.

According to the Bureau of Labor Statistics, in March 2010 the cost per pound of chicken breast, bone-in and boneless, was $2.25 and $3.26 respectively, and the cost of dried beans per pound was $1.36. Buying a pound of beans instead of a pound of chicken would cost you $0.89 to $1.90 less, and a pound of beans will feed you for more meals than a pound of chicken will. In the same month, rice was $0.76 per pound, apples were $1.17 per pound, bananas were $0.56 per pound, and lettuce was $0.86 per pound. Contrast this with $3.10 per pound for ground beef, $5.29 per pound for steaks, and $2.28 per pound for ham.

There's really no question that you can eat more cheaply on a plant-based diet than on a meat-based one. In fact, that's the initial reason many college students try a vegetarian diet. But in the end, leaning in to vegetarian fare isn't only about saving money at the grocery store. There are so many hidden costs to eating meat—from how it makes us feel to the diseases it promotes to the environment and our fellow creatures. The production of meat is a direct cause of climate change (see Promise 6), the annual cost of which in the U.S. alone is expected to reach more than $2 trillion. The Natural Resources Defense Council recently published a report by Tufts University climate scientists indicating that "four global warming impacts alone—hurricane damage, real estate losses, energy costs, and water costs—will come with a price tag of . . . almost $1.9 trillion annually (in today's dollars) by 2100." Animal waste pollutes our waterways, workers are made sick both physically and psychologically by working in slaughterhouses and CAFOs, and we are sickened, too.

It's easy to see that the hidden costs of eating meat are everywhere—in how you feel day to day, in your prospects for a long life of good health, in the health of the land, the water, the animals, the workers, . . . and your pocketbook. It's pretty compelling, isn't it?

Becoming a veganist is about very consciously choosing to disengage from an industry that makes us sick, abuses animals, pollutes the planet, and squanders precious resources. It's also about a better quality of life—having more energy and a lighter load (as well as a lighter conscience) and living longer and healthier.

And that's not something that can be measured in dollars and cents.

You Will Radically Reduce Your Carbon Footprint and Do the Single Best Thing You Can for the Environment

Did you know?

- The business of raising animals for food (with its continuous heavy waste stream of methane and nitrous oxide—leading global warming gases) is responsible for about 18 percent of global warming.
- Animal agriculture takes up an incredible 70 percent of all agricultural land, and a whopping 30 percent of the land surface of the planet.
- As a result, farmed animals are probably the biggest cause of slashing and burning of the world's forests.
- The United States' most influential environmental group—Environmental Defense Fund—has calculated that if every American skipped

one meal of chicken per week and substituted vegetarian foods, the carbon dioxide savings would be the same as if the nation removed more than half a million cars from U.S. roads.

- **A person prevents more climate change pollution by going vegetarian than by switching to a hybrid car.**
- **It takes, on average, more than ten times as much fossil fuel to make one calorie of animal protein as it does to make one calorie of plant protein.**

A few years ago, the environmental journalist Paul Hawken challenged students from the University of Portland with a thought experiment:

Ralph Waldo Emerson once asked what we would do if the stars only came out once every thousand years. No one would sleep that night, of course. The world would create new religions overnight. We would be ecstatic, delirious, made rapturous by the glory of God. Instead the stars come out every night, and we watch television.

This extraordinary time when we are globally aware of each other and the multiple dangers that threaten civilization has never happened, not in a thousand years, not in ten thousand years. Each of us is as complex and beautiful as all the stars in the universe. We have done great things and we have gone way off course in terms of honoring creation. You are graduating to the most amazing, stupefying challenge ever bequested to any generation. The generations before you failed. They didn't stay up all night. They got distracted and lost sight of the fact that life is a miracle every moment of your existence. Nature beckons you to be on her side. You couldn't ask for a better boss. The most unrealistic person in the world is the cynic, not the dreamer. Hope only makes sense when it doesn't make sense to be hopeful. This is your century. Take it and run, *as if your life depends on it.*

We all know it so clearly that it almost seems silly to say it: our planet is in trouble. But it's also critically important to say it—perhaps it's more important than anything else, since so many profit so much from our forgetting. We need only check the news for a few days, and it's painfully obvious that Hawken is right in his analysis: As I type, the East Coast is getting ready for the worst storms in decades, and we've just survived the craziest winter weather ever recorded— and both events, within a few months of one another in the exact same ecosystem, are directly attributable to climate change.

Everywhere, water is drying up and getting filthier, fires are burning out of control because of hotter temperatures and drought-ridden brush; fish are disappearing (and with them goes the food chain), storms are getting wilder, species are becoming extinct, and the very air itself is making some of us sick. Again, Hawken is right: Time is running out. The time to act is now.

The good news is that we can tilt things in a better direction by shifting the way we eat. It turns out that the single most potent thing we, as individuals, can do for the planet's well-being is to eat a more plant-based diet. More than changing your lightbulbs, or driving a hybrid car, or turning down the heat, you can do better by the environment by cutting back on animal-based food.

Think of it this way: Just like humans, animals have to eat to survive. You probably consume between 1,200 and 2,500 calories per day, depending on your size, the nature of your job, and how much time you spend exercising. And you burn all those calories off, simply existing. Farmed animals, also, burn the vast majority of their caloric intake off keeping their bodies going. And then some significant portion of their caloric intake produces feathers, skin, blood, and other parts of their bodies that we don't consume. Once you crunch the numbers, you find that feeding animals for meat, dairy, and egg production requires growing some ten times as many crops as we'd need if we just ate pasta primavera, veggie sausage, and other plant based foods directly (rather than funneling those crops through animals).

On top of this inherent vast inefficiency of the animal foods industries, we also have to transport the animals to slaughterhouses, slaughter them, refrigerate their carcasses, and distribute their flesh all across the country. Producing a calorie of meat protein means burning more than ten times, on average, as much fossil fuel (with all the greenhouse gas emissions and other pollution that entails) as producing a calorie of plant protein does.

Plus, animal agriculture takes up an incredible 70 percent of all agricultural land, and a whopping 30 percent of the land surface of the planet. As a result, farmed animals are probably the biggest cause of slashing and burning of the world's forests. (More than 95 percent of soy is fed to animals—not human beings.) Today, 70 percent of former Amazon rain forest is used for pastureland, and feed crops cover much of the remainder. These forests serve as "sinks" and are often referred to as the lungs of the planet, absorbing carbon dioxide from the air, so turning these forests into soy fields so that those of us in the first world can have cheap chicken releases all that stored carbon dioxide, further warming the planet.

The Intergovernmental Panel on Climate Change, which won the Nobel Peace Prize for working to raise global consciousness about the issue of climate change, has described the existence of human-caused global warming in its final assessment report as both "unequivocal," and as having "abrupt and irreversible" effects on global climate. Worse still, these effects are coming stronger and faster than predicted in the panel's most recent report. Alarmingly, some effects that had been expected to arrive decades from now are already here.

The report warns that hundreds of millions of people are threatened with starvation, flooding, and weather disasters. Rain-fed crop production will fall by half, a quarter of the world's species will go extinct, and some arctic ice will completely disappear during the summer. We will see more deadly heat waves, stronger hurricanes, and island nations completely obliterated by rising sea levels. It sounds biblical in proportion, and even though the most severe effects have not been directly experienced by most of us yet, things do appear to be getting worse, year by storm-drenched year.

On the issue of climate change, animal agriculture is a nightmare in comparison to producing grains and beans and other plant-based foods. In a 400-page report from the United Nations' Food and Agricultural Organization, "Livestock's Long Shadow," UN agricultural scientists conclude that the business of raising animals for food is responsible for about 18 percent of all warming, and that meat eating is "one of the top two or three most significant contributors to the most serious environmental problems, at every scale from local to global." World Bank agricultural scientists rebutted the UN in 2010, arguing that, actually, the number is not 18 percent, but rather at least 50 percent. The most highly esteemed agricultural scientists are saying that animal agriculture is at least one half of the problem of climate change.

It's a little hard to fathom when you think about a small chick hatching from her fragile egg. How can an animal, so seemingly insignificant against the vastness of the earth, give off enough greenhouse gas to change the global climate? The answer is in their sheer numbers. We slaughter around 10 billion land animals a year in this country alone, and *60 billion* are slaughtered worldwide. Remember that all these animals have to eat—feed mills have to operate, trucks have to tote the feed (and the animals and their carcasses) from here to there. And on and on—producing massive amounts of carbon dioxide (CO_2). But that's not the only warming gas that worries scientists.

Carbon dioxide counts for about half of global warming

gases, and a third is from methane and nitrous oxide. These superstrong gases come primarily from farmed animals' digestive processes and from their manure. In fact, while animal agriculture accounts for 9 percent of our carbon dioxide emissions, it emits 37 percent of our methane, and a whopping 65 percent of our nitrous oxide. Methane is twenty times as powerful as CO_2 as a planet warmer, and N_{20} is almost 300 times as powerful. By simply raising fewer (or no) animals, we could turn off these climate change spigots.

What we're seeing is just the beginning, too. Meat consumption has increased fivefold in the past fifty years, and is expected to double again in the next fifty, encouraged by growing global affluence and enormous advertising campaigns by the animal agriculture companies that tell us to drink more milk and eat more meat. We are not only eating ourselves to death, but we are also eating our planet to death.

I often hear people say, "I don't eat red meat because I know cows give off methane." But the factory farming of chickens releases tremendous amounts of greenhouse gas emissions as well. Industrial farming of any animals is a problem because, whether for cows, pigs, or chickens, food still has to be grown and turned into animal feed, and extra trucks and factories are operated that would not be needed for plant foods. So if you do indeed decide to cut back on meat, cut back on all meat, because just switching from beef to chicken doesn't make much of a difference.

And it's not just a matter of global warming gases: with chickens, as with pigs and cattle, vast quantities of dangerous chemicals are produced, acidic and tainted urine seeps into the groundwater, and bacteria-laden manure infects the soil, thanks to concentrated animal-feeding operations.

In a story about chicken-waste pollution, the *New York Times* reported that "[a]lthough the dairy and hog industry in states near the bay produce more pounds of manure, poultry waste has more than twice the concentration of pollutants per pound." That's probably in part because calorie for calorie, chickens are given a lot more drugs than pigs and cattle—because they're kept in even worse conditions.

When you have the attorney general of a state like Oklahoma battling poultry producers over the industry "wreak[ing] havoc in the 1-million-acre Illinois River watershed, turning it into a murky, sludgy mess" (Associated Press, 2008), it seems pretty clear that all meat—whether from cattle, pigs, or chickens—is a big problem for the environment. There is just no way to raise billions of animals without compromising the environment in myriad ways.

As I struggle to figure out what to include—and what not to include—in this chapter, I am struck by the sheer enormity of the problem. Remember, that UN report is more than 400 pages long. It concludes that meat production contributes to "problems of land degradation, global warming and air pollution, water shortage and water pollution, and loss of biodiversity." Similarly, books like John Robbins's

The Food Revolution devote hundreds of pages to the issue of farmed animal waste and pollution. Please take a close look into those two sources; the information therein is just stunning.

From the United Nations' Food and Agricultural Organization, "Livestock's Long Shadow": eating meat is "one of the most significant contributors to the most serious environmental problems, at every scale from local to global."

I'll close out this discussion of farmed animal waste and pollution with these few additional facts: Animal agriculture accounts for most of the water consumed in this country, emits two-thirds of the world's acid-rain-causing ammonia, and is the world's largest source of water pollution—killing entire river and marine ecosystems, destroying coral reefs, and of course, making people sick. Try to imagine the prodigious volumes of manure churned out by modern American farms: 5 million tons a day, more than three times the fecal waste of the human population, and far more than our land can possibly absorb. The acres and acres of cesspools stretching over much of our countryside, polluting the air and contaminating our water, make the *Exxon Valdez* oil spill look minor in comparison.

Trawlers each as long as a football field clear-cut the
ocean floor and can take in 800,000 pounds of fish in
a single outing.

I do, however, want to say a few words about the most
neglected of all animals we eat: sea animals. Fishing, like
farming, isn't what it used to be. This fact was most clearly
hammered home for me when I saw a video that Sir Paul
McCartney put out called *Glass Walls*. McCartney is probably the West's most famous and outspoken vegetarian, and
the title comes from the fact that, apparently, Sir Paul is always telling people, "If slaughterhouses had glass walls,
everyone would be a vegetarian." Anyway, I have seen quite
a few videos—including undercover investigations—that
document the cruelties of factory farms, but I had not seen
much on the fish industry. Sir Paul's video (which you can
find easily with an Internet search of his name and "Glass
Walls") opened my eyes, and I can't recommend it highly
enough.

Trawlers each as long as a football field clear-cut the
ocean floor and can take in 800,000 pounds of fish in a single outing. Obviously, they are scooping up anything and
everything that is in their path: dolphins, turtles, and coral
reefs get scraped up and destroyed right along with whatever
the boat was actually trying to catch. Large chunks of the
ocean floor are dredged up as about 30 million tons of dead
sea animals (called bycatch) along with fatally injured

creatures of all sorts, are tossed back overboard (throwing delicate aquatic ecosystems into disarray). As a result of the growing demand for fish, the populations of some of the most common fish species have dropped by 90 percent in the past fifty years.

And farmed fish is even worse, because it requires about five pounds of wild-caught fish to reap one pound of farmed fish. *Huh?* I hear you cry. It *what?* As with so much about the meat industry, this reality blows my mind, too. You see, because our oceans are being destroyed, the most desirable fish for human consumption are now, to a huge degree, farmed. The fish the trawlers catch are, often, fish that are less marketable.

The solution? In a twist worthy of George Orwell, the wild-caught fish are fed to the farmed fish, so that, voilà: farmed fish actually cause more deep-sea trawling than, even, the market for wild-caught fish. Are you confused yet? Read it again: It will never make sense, but after a few reads, you'll likely see that anyone concerned about the environment might consider leaving fish off their diet.

I'm sure everything I've just recounted sounds like cause for despair, but in fact, there's another way of looking at it. Remember Paul Hawken's challenge at the University of Portland? He continued with words that are deeply relevant to our discussion. He challenged his listeners, "Forget that this task of planet-saving is not possible in the time required. Don't be put off by people who know what is not possible. Do what needs to be done, and check to see if it was impossible only after you are done." Sure, things are bad. But we have the power to change it all. We have a powerful new weapon to use against the most serious environmental crisis ever to face humanity. Now that we know a greener diet is even more effective than a greener car (vegan is the new Prius!), we can make a difference at every single meal, simply by leaving the animals off of our plates. We can fix so much of this mess with surprising ease, just by putting down our chicken wings and reaching for a veggie burger instead.

CHEW ON THIS!

Excrement produced by livestock: **14 billion tons per year, more than a million pounds per second—** that's sixty times as much as produced by the world's human population—more in one day than the U.S. human population produces in three and a half years.

Water used for livestock and irrigating feed crops: **240 trillion gallons per day—7.5 million gallons per second—** that's enough for every human to take eight showers a day, or as much as used each day by Europe, Africa, and South America combined.

Soil erosion due to growing livestock feed: **40 billion tons per year**

Land used to raise animals for food: **10 billion acres**

If every American skipped one meal of chicken per week and substituted vegetarian foods instead, the carbon dioxide savings would be the same as taking more than half a million cars off U.S. roads.

"About 20 percent of the world's pastures and rangelands, with 73 percent of rangelands in dry areas, have been degraded to some extent, mostly through overgrazing, compaction and erosion created by livestock action." (UN)

Crops raised for livestock feed that could otherwise feed people: **1 billion tons per year—63,000 pounds per second**

Emissions of greenhouse gases from raising animals for food: **The equivalent of 7.1 billion metric tons of carbon dioxide per year**

"The livestock sector is . . . responsible for 18 percent of greenhouse gas emissions." (UN)

It takes more than ten times as much fossil fuel to make one calorie of animal protein as it does to make one calorie of plant protein.

An American saves more global warming pollution by going vegetarian than by switching their car to a hybrid Prius.

Former Amazon rainforest converted to raising animals for food since 1970 amounts to more than 90 percent of all Amazon deforestation since 1970.

"Livestock now account for about 20 percent of the total terrestrial animal biomass, and the 30 percent of the earth's land surface that they now pre-empt was once habitat for wildlife." (UN)

If everyone went vegetarian for just one day, the U.S. would save:

- 100 billion gallons of water, enough to supply all the homes in New England for almost 4 months;
- 1.5 billion pounds of crops otherwise fed to livestock, enough to feed the state of New Mexico for more than a year;
- 70 million gallons of gas—enough to fuel all the cars of Canada and Mexico combined with plenty to spare;
- 3 million acres of land, an area more than twice the size of Delaware;
- 33 tons of antibiotics.

If everyone went vegetarian for just one day, the U.S. would prevent:

- Greenhouse gas emissions equivalent to 1.2 million tons of CO_2, as much as is produced by all of France in a single day;
- 3 million tons of soil erosion and $70 million in resulting economic damages;
- 4.5 million tons of animal excrement;
- Almost 7 tons of ammonia emissions, a major air pollutant.

Sources: "Livestock's Long Shadow" (United Nations), the World Bank, and calculations of Noam Mohr, a physicist at the Polytechnic Institute of New York University.

PROMISE 7:

You Will Be Helping Provide Food to the Global Poor

Did you know?

- Approximately 1 billion people—⅙ of the population—on this planet don't have enough to eat.
- 40 percent of the world's grain goes to feeding livestock.
- In the year 2007 alone, approximately 100 million metric tons of grain and corn was turned into biofuels, which in turn drove up food prices for the global poor by 75 percent, according to a World Bank report; in that same period, 756 million metric tons was fed to chickens, pigs, and other farmed animals.
- If 1 in 10 people around the globe stopped eating animals, it would free up enough food to feed the 1 billion hungry.

Try and wrap your head around this: Right now, approximately a billion people on this planet don't have enough to eat. That is nearly a sixth of the world's population. That's right. One out of every six of our fellow humans has to scrounge for food and feel the ache of an empty stomach every day. And each and every year, tens of millions (15 million of them children) die from starvation-related problems like infections and diarrhea—all this even as Americans get more and more obese.

In fact, in a report by Worldwatch Institute called *Underfed and Overfed* their scientists note that 1.2 billion people in the world are underfed and malnourished, while approximately the same number, a different group of 1.2 billion people, are *over*fed and malnourished. And both the hungry and the overweight have high levels of sickness, shortened life expectancies, and lower levels of productivity, albeit for entirely opposite reasons—the overfed tend to die of cancer, heart disease, and diabetes while the underfed tend to die of infectious diseases and waterborne illnesses.

As Americans get more and more obese, tens of millions (15 million of them children) around the world die from malnutrition, infection, and diarrhea.

In another report by Worldwatch called *State of the World*, it was noted that 56 percent of the children in Bangladesh are underfed and underweight to the point of illness; in the same report they also found that 55 percent of adults in the U.S. are so overfed and overweight that *their* health is diminished. The imbalance in food distribution and availability is causing serious problems on both sides of the spectrum. How did this happen?

When I was growing up, my mother used to chide me to finish the dinner on my plate, saying that there were starving people in Africa, and that it was shameful to leave food uneaten. I didn't quite understand how forcing myself to swallow the last bits of grizzled chicken or beef was being respectful to poor and hungry children in developing countries, but I did what I was told. Instead of feeling like I did the right thing, though, I had a gnawing sense that something was askew. Years later when I read Frances Moore Lappé's book *Diet for a Small Planet*, I realized that in my earnest desire to do the right thing by the global poor, I was in fact supporting the very hunger I felt so badly about. Here's why . . .

When you eat meat, it's like you are taking food right out of the mouths of the poor. The grain that could have fed hungry people instead is shipped to factory farms to feed the 10 billion animals (in the U.S. alone) who are being fattened up for profitable slaughter.

In order for cows, chickens, and pigs to grow big and fat (and fetch a higher price on the market) they of course have to eat. And eat a lot. They are fed feed that is predominantly composed of corn and soy (grown in the U.S. as well as in developing countries) to make them as big as possible, as quickly as possible. Much of the grain they eat goes just to keeping them alive—breathing, building blood and bone, and repairing tissue—rather than forming edible muscle meat. Of course cows are not designed to eat grains; their natural diet is grasses. (But that's a whole 'nother subject . . .)

It takes many pounds of grain to create just one pound of meat—more than 16 to 1 in the case of beef. Put another way, a quantity of grain that could feed fifty people creates just *one* 8-ounce steak, a "small" steak by some standards.

Essentially, as long as the animal agriculture industry is willing to pay more than developing nations for the grain used to feed their animals, the global poor will suffer. In fact, 40 percent of the world's grain goes to feeding livestock. People in developing countries simply cannot match the prices paid by more affluent countries, with their insatiable appetites for meat. And it's not only the grain that gets wasted on feeding livestock; water and soil here and abroad are being used at that same wasteful rate. Instead of growing food for subsistence in their own backyards, the world's poor are starving while farming cash crops to send abroad. Simply put, our addiction to meat has created an imbalance in the distribution and availability of food. A plant-based diet would reduce our reliance on a system of trade that is harmful to the global poor.

If you've been alert to this debate at all, you've probably heard that the grain fed to farmed animals is feed grain, not food grain. While that might be technically correct, the land, water, fuel, and all the other resources that go into raising crops which feed livestock could instead be used to grow food grains that are suitable for humans. It is an easy and sensible switch to make.

You might also hear that grazing animals eat grasses that cannot be consumed by humans, thereby serving as an intrinsic link in making food fit for human consumption by converting the vegetation into edible protein (animal flesh); but for the developed world, this is the very definition of a specious argument: It sounds good, but it falls flat under even the most cursory scrutiny. In the United States, more than 95 percent of pigs, chickens, and turkeys never spend any time in pasture, even though these animals were built for greens. The only animals who spend any significant amount of time grazing are cattle (about six months), and even they are crammed together in feedlots for more than half their lives, where they are fed vast quantities of animal feed. It is the business of these factory farms to get the animals as fat as possible as quickly as possible, and this is accomplished by keeping them indoors gorging on animal feed.

The Biofuel Connection

There is a direct and measurable relationship between human starvation and the grain being grown for industry. A few years ago, the UN's special envoy on food, Jean Ziegler, decried the growing production of biofuels: While human beings are starving, he argued, it is a crime against humanity that grains and corn would be converted into fuel. He has a point: According to the UN, in 2007 approximately 100 million metric tons of grain and corn was turned into biofuels.

Biofuels have driven up food prices for the global poor by 75 percent, according to a World Bank report. The *Guardian*'s coverage of the report notes that "[r]ising food prices have pushed 100 [million] people worldwide below the poverty line . . . and have sparked riots from Bangladesh to Egypt."

The thing is, more than *756* million metric tons of grain and corn were fed to farmed animals in the same year, as was almost all the global soy crop (approximately 220 million metric tons). In our global marketplace, if you choose to eat chicken, you are (in a very real way) a part of a macroeconomic system that causes a billion people to go hungry for want of any food at all. The Worldwatch Institute puts it this way: "[M]eat consumption is an inefficient use of grain—the grain is used more efficiently when consumed by humans. Continued growth in meat output is dependent on feeding grain to animals, creating competition for grain between affluent meat-eaters and the world's poor."

To compound the problem, as countries like China and India become wealthier, there is an increasing demand for meat because meat is seen as a status symbol; meat seems to represent wealth because those who are poor cannot afford it. One of my best friends is Chinese, and she tells me how, when she was young and living in a humble village in the country-side a few hours outside Beijing, she and her family would enjoy a once-a-year feast of a pig's head roasted over a pit. They couldn't afford the choicer cuts of the animal, but always dreamed of one day being able to eat more and "better" meat like they saw rich people do.

Now that she and her family have moved definitively out of that class, it's hard for my friend to make sense of going back to the way she ate in childhood—mostly a plant-based diet of rice, soy, and vegetables with only a tiny little bit of meat or fish as garnish or flavoring. She didn't want to eat what she thought was a peasant's diet now that she had "arrived," so meat became the main event at every meal. (I have since disabused her of the notion that a plant-based diet is associated with deprivation or asceticism!) So as more and more previously poor people enter the middle class, more animals will be raised for their newly acquired tastes and budgets, which exponentially undermines the efforts of the remaining global poor to be able to feed themselves.

Even Peter R. Cheeke, an industry expert and a professor of animal agriculture at Oregon State University acknowledges, "Beef has become a symbol of the extravagant, resource-consuming American who is destroying the global environment to live a life of luxury, while most of the rest of the world suffer pestilence and famine. . . . Strictly on a scientific basis, there can be no dispute that corn and soybean meal are used with more efficiency, and can provide food for more people, when they are eaten directly by people rather than being fed to swine or poultry to be converted to pork, chicken meat, or eggs for human consumption."

And how about this amazing statistic: if one in ten people around the globe stopped eating animals, it would free up enough food to feed the one billion hungry—so says a report called *Feeding the Future*, by the National Library of Medicine at the National Institutes of Health.

Why should we care about all this? After all, anyone reading this book is likely living in a wealthy country with plenty to eat. Most of us hopefully have a sincere desire to see everyone do well and thrive, whether they live near us and within our communities or not. We want to see the scourge of hunger and poverty end, but short of sending money through organizations to people in need, we don't quite know how to make a meaningful difference. But when we change our diet to reflect our values—for example, the belief that food is a basic human right—we feel like we are on track with our better instincts.

By cutting back on or forgoing meat, dairy, fish, and eggs in favor of a plant-based diet, we say no to a system that makes it ever more difficult for poor people to feed themselves. We know that we can't have peace in the world—or in our souls, for that matter—if any one of us is starving.

And isn't it just perfect that the very diet that can help to eradicate hunger can also prevent and reverse the most serious of our modern diseases, turn around environmental disaster, and lessen the suffering of billions of animals?

PROMISE 8:

You Will Reduce
Animal Suffering

Did you know?

- The vast majority—over 95 percent—of animals are raised in factory farms and not on the old-fashioned family farms of memory.

- In typical egg-producing operations, egg-laying hens are crammed by the bunch into tiny wire cages stacked one upon the other for hundreds of yards. They cannot spread their wings, and they are often piled on top of each other; sometimes with broken bones, open sores, and feather loss.

- Broiler chickens, which make up 8.5 of the nearly 10 billion animals raised for food each year, are often drugged up and genetically manipulated to grow extremely large, extremely quickly, and as a result they often cannot support their unnatural weight—their legs remain malformed or break. Their hearts and lungs cannot keep up with the unnaturally rapid growth, and many die of heart or lung failure.

- When stunners aren't effective, hogs are sometimes sent into the scalding tanks, meant to soften the skin of dead pigs, while they are still alive and conscious.

- Cattle often have their horns ripped out, are castrated and branded without painkillers, and end up standing in their own filth for months before they're slaughtered. Because the rate of kills is typically up to 400 animals per hour, the line is not stopped if the stun gun is not effective—thus, animals may be dismembered while still alive.

More and more people are choosing to lean toward a plant-based diet out of a desire not to do harm to animals. That was most certainly what got me to think about what I was eating. I had put off for many years reading a few books about animals and food that I knew would change me forever. But once I started reading accounts and watching videos about what happened to animals as they made their way to my plate, I was consumed with the idea that there had to be a better way. It makes a huge statement—to forgo meat to reduce suffering. And it feels great to know that your food choices cause little to no harm.

In this chapter we're going to look squarely at the way animals are raised for food. Let me say from the outset that this chapter will be *hard* to read. It was also the hardest for me to write. The reality is ugly, and not only is there no way to sugarcoat it, but it would be terribly irresponsible of me to avoid the subject or gloss over it. The way animals are raised and treated is, in a word, indefensible. If you are not already convinced, perhaps you will be, once you know all the facts about what goes on behind the scenes.

For this chapter I spoke with many people who have seen animal agriculture from the inside. You'll hear directly from several of them. Let's just say there is a reason you can't simply peer into the windows of slaughterhouses, why they're in out-of-the-way places and aren't made of glass.

My friend Bruce Wieland told me the following story about growing up on a farm, and how he came to realize that a plant-based diet was right for him.

Bruce Wieland's Story:
A Journey Begins

I grew up on a farm in South Texas and I was five years old the first time I saw an animal slaughtered. It was November and the first norther of the season had arrived overnight, sending the temperatures down into the high forties. It had been hot the day before, and when I woke up that morning I was excited by the sudden change in the weather.

Cold weather meant the holidays were coming. It meant my mother would be baking cakes and cinnamon rolls. We would be getting a Christmas tree soon. It also meant I would finally be able to wear my "new" winter coat. It wasn't really new. It was a hand-me-down from one of my older brothers who had long outgrown it. The coat was gray twill with a thick cotton fleece lining. It had a hood, deep pockets, a zipper in the front, and I thought it made me look very grown up. I had been trying it on for months, looking forward to having a legitimate reason to wear it, and now, at last, the first norther had arrived. It was the perfect weather for a new coat.

As it turned out, it was also the perfect weather for butchering a hog. On butcher days, my mother would close off the workroom from the rest of the house and open the doors and windows to let in the cold air, allowing us to work indoors with the meat without it spoiling. All this I learned about later. That particular morning in November, I was just excited about the cold weather and wearing my coat. My father was getting ready to go outside. He put on his heavy boots, his jacket, his winter cap, and got his .22 rifle out of the gun closet. When I asked if I could go with him, he said yes, but my mother looked at him disapprovingly and turned to me saying no, she was sure this was not something I would want to see. I don't remember how long they discussed it, but my mother was eventually outvoted two to one. She reluctantly pulled my hood up over my head and tied it under my chin. As my dad and I walked out the back door, my mother told him to be careful and to make sure I was safely out of the way. That made it sound dangerous, which I thought was exciting, and I remember walking down to the hog pens happy to be going on an adventure.

At some point, I'm sure my father explained what was going to happen. He must have told me he was going to shoot a pig so we could make sausage and have bacon and pork chops, which I liked. But all I really remember about our walk is the cold air and the wet grass and feeling snug and safe and warm in my gray coat.

The hog pens were on two large concrete slabs that were tilted slightly to allow the manure to be easily hosed into a central trough that drained into a nearby cesspool. There were six pens in all, separated by horizontal metal pipes welded to upright metal posts. My father handed me the rifle to hold while he climbed over the bars into one of the pens, where there were about a dozen young pigs. Once he was inside, I handed him the rifle and he pulled me up onto the edge of the slab where I could hold onto the bars from the outside and see into the pen.

They were only three or four months old, nowhere near full grown. I was struck by how evident their different personalities were. Some were playing, running around each other in circles. They would press against one another, then do a little trick where one pig would stick her snout under the belly of another pig and lift him up an inch or so then turn and run, and the pig who had been lifted would chase after her like they were playing tag. Two or three pigs, however, stood perfectly still, watching my father's every move as though they were aware that something was different about this morning. Most of them, though, thinking they were about to be fed, gathered around my father, who looked them over carefully then pointed to one of the pigs who was nuzzling his leg for food, and said, I think this is the one we want.

Using the barrel of the rifle, he gently tapped the pig on his shoulders, guiding him away from the other pigs toward the corner of the pen nearest where I was standing. To me, the pig seemed to think this was some kind of game he was eager to play but didn't quite understand. With each tap, he would take a step forward then look back over his shoulder at my father, as though to check to see if he was doing it right. After a few more steps, when the pig was in the right position facing into the corner a few feet from where I was standing, my father glanced over to make sure I was watching, then he moved the muzzle of the gun to the back of the pig's head. The pig tilted his head slightly and looked up at me. He gave a little grunt. My father pulled the trigger.

The bullet shattered the pig's forehead on its exit and sent a fine splattering of blood into the air. I blinked when I felt the warm mist on my face and hands. When I opened my eyes, I saw the pig lying on his side and a thick stream of blood running from his head down the slanted concrete. The other pigs had scrambled for the opposite corner and were squealing and climbing on top of each other trying to get as far away as possible. My father knelt to make sure the pig was dead, then looked up for my reaction. I'm sure his heart stopped a moment when he saw me. I was covered with tiny drops of blood. He jumped out of the pen, lifted me off the slab and carried me to a water faucet where he wet his handkerchief, wiped the blood off my face, and washed my hands under the cold running water.

I remember that he was talking, but I don't remember anything he said. I pulled away from him and started walking back to the house. He called, but I didn't answer. Instead, I started running. I was again aware of the wet grass and the cold air, and I kept thinking that just a few minutes earlier, the blood on my coat had been inside the pig and he had been alive and happy and walking around with his friends, thinking he was going to get something to eat. And now he was dead with his head blown open and his blood running down the slab, and all this had happened because of me—because I wanted to go outside wearing my coat. Later, when I confessed this to my parents, they told me that the pig would have been killed whether I had been there or not. I did not find that comforting and I did not believe them.

My mother washed the blood out of the gray jacket, but I never wore it again. I had changed. I was now aware that I lived in a place where animals were killed. I never walked by the cement slab without remembering that pig, the first of thousands of animals I saw butchered or loaded up for transport to the slaughterhouse. It never got easier to watch. It was never okay with me and I could never understand why it didn't seem to bother anyone else. My parents often said that they didn't enjoy killing animals, but they had to because that's how we got our food. I was taught in school that eating meat was essential for good health, and since every single person I knew and loved did it, how could it be wrong?

It took years to unravel and correct all the misperceptions and misinformation from my childhood. In time, I learned that my family's hog operation was idyllic compared with what happens on today's factory farms and in modern slaughterhouses, where death is neither quick nor painless. As I became more interested in farmed-animal welfare, I watched many videos. One in particular still haunts me. It showed an endless stream of pigs, each hanging by one of their back legs on hooks attached to a moving track, like clothes at a dry cleaner. The pigs were screaming and struggling to free themselves as one by one, the workers slit open the veins in their necks and began hacking them apart, some while they were visibly still alive and conscious, their eyes bulging, their expressive faces twisted in agony, fear, and confusion.

Pigs are intelligent, highly social animals with personalities as complex and unique as any cat or dog. But that doesn't stop us from killing 115 million of them every year.

My journey into this awareness of animals began with the killing of a small white pig on that chilly November morning. With that experience, I learned to doubt, and eventually, to challenge, the status quo and to ask questions, all of which were variations on the one question no one could answer: If killing animals for food is necessary and right, why in my heart and soul does it feel so deeply wrong?

I stopped eating meat when I was twenty-four years old. My only regret is that I didn't do it sooner. I'm fifty now, and when I consider all the choices I've made in my life, I can say without hesitation that the choice to stop eating meat is by far the single best decision I've ever made.

It was effortless. I was ready. I had been ready since I was five.

My friend Gene Baur, one of the founders of the New York State–based organization Farm Sanctuary, has also seen a lot. He goes to factory farms and tries to rescue animals who have been discarded because they can't walk or are not in shape to be profitable. Here's a story he recently told me.

Gene Baur's Story:
The Rescuer

I visited this veal farm several times, documenting how calves were chained by the neck unable to walk or even turn around. They lived in a dark windowless shed. Over the weeks, the calves grew larger, and became increasingly cramped and frustrated by their confinement. One day, I went back to the farm and found the crates empty because the calves had been sent to slaughter. But one calf was too sick to walk onto the slaughterhouse truck and had collapsed in the alleyway, where he was left to die. The calf was on his side and not able to lift his head. When I stepped in front of him, he looked at me. There was fear in his eyes, and he probably didn't want to ever see a human being again. It was such an eerie moment; the calf was so quiet. The whole barn was quiet and empty. The animals that had been confined there for months were gone, except for this one calf left in the alleyway. I believed I could help him, and called law enforcement; but he didn't make it. I am constantly haunted by what I can't do, but try not to focus on it.

At hatcheries that hatch egg-laying hens, millions of unwanted male chicks are discarded every year because they're of no economic value—they don't grow fast enough to be raised profitably for meat, and they'll never lay eggs. I've seen Dumpsters filled with thousands of dead and dying male chicks; and I've also seen these day-old hatchlings dumped into a manure spreader to be put out on the field like fertilizer. I could hear faint chirping sounds coming from the manure spreader. Several chicks were trying to survive, perched on debris in the spreader, trying not to drown in the muck. I am struck by the irony of baby chicks, symbols of spring and new life, being killed immediately after emerging from their shells.

When documenting conditions at a Texas stockyard, I saw this cow in a pen, with her head flopped over to one side. I asked the stockyard worker what happened and was told that the cow was brought to the stockyard with her calf, and they were forcibly separated as is common in the cattle industry. Cows have very close bonds with their young, and when mother and calf are separated—usually at day one—the mother bellows and cries for hours and sometimes days. This mother fought to be with her calf, but she was restrained and couldn't go after him as he was dragged away. When she lunged toward him, someone slammed the gate on her and her neck was broken. Her eyes were wide open, full of fear, moving and darting around. Sometimes her head would swing wildly across the floor, but she couldn't lift it. There was actually a groove in the pen where her head had swung back and forth. I felt sick and pained and helpless. She was to be used for meat, so there was little chance she would be put out of her misery.

And here is an account by Josh Balk, who now works at the Humane Society of the United States.

Josh Balk's Story:
Undercover at a Chicken Factory

In September 2004, on behalf of the organization Compassion over Killing, I got a job working undercover for a few weeks at a chicken slaughter plant. While I had seen plenty of animal slaughter footage, I had never experienced how truly horrific and heartbreaking the process was until I witnessed it firsthand as an employee at this plant.

My first day working at the plant was spent filling out forms, watching videos, and listening to presentations. At no time did anyone mention animal welfare, nor did trainers ever provide me any guidance on "proper animal handling." In fact, during several hours of videos, there were only about three seconds of footage of live animals, and that was during a montage of different activities that require workers to lift objects.

My second day began in the live hang room, where workers shackle chickens onto the slaughter line. As soon as I entered the room, the smell of chicken waste hit me so hard that I struggled to keep myself from vomiting. The line leader led me to my position on the line and gave me only one sentence of instruction: "Pick up the chickens upside down and put their legs in the shackles." With that, he walked away. I was on my own.

Speed was the most important objective, since our workday ended once a quota was achieved. Workers grabbed the chickens as quickly—and thereby as roughly—as possible from the conveyor belt, often picking them up by one wing, one leg, or their necks. They often forced the chickens into the metal shackles so hard, I was amazed their legs weren't ripped off. Although the birds were supposed to be hung upside down by both legs, sometimes they dangled by just one.

After only thirty minutes of working on the line, two things stood out more than anything else: how the animals were treated and how they reacted.

Many of the chickens responded with screams and violent physical reactions from the moment the workers grabbed them. The screaming, frenzied wing flapping, and drone of the heavy machinery were so loud that you had to yell to the worker next to you, who was less than two feet away, just so he could hear you.

Workers didn't just treat the animals aggressively while they were hanging them. I saw an employee kick a chicken off the floor fan and routinely saw, and of course secretly videotaped, workers throwing chickens around the room. Some birds managed to jump from the conveyor belt onto the floor before they were shackled, so workers would grab them and throw them back toward the belt. A couple of times, workers threw the chickens so hard, the entire line shook from the force of their bodies hitting the shackles.

All the chickens I saw had severe feather loss on their stomachs and chests, presumably ammonia burns from living and lying in their own waste in the "grow-out" facility. Poultry companies breed chickens to grow large so quickly: by the end of their life they're often unable even to stand or walk for any significant period of time, thus they're relegated to lying down for the vast majority of the day.

At one point during my employment, so many chickens had piled up on top of each other at one end of the conveyor belt, the line backed up. The worker on that end quickly grabbed the chickens and threw them back down the line to clear the conveyor entrance of birds. One of the birds was thrown right past my face, nearly hitting me. Neither the supervisor nor any of the other workers said anything to the employee throwing the chickens. All I heard from one worker was, "Let's go! Hurry up!"

While working there I tried to hang the birds as gently as possible, which made me slower than my co-workers. The supervisor saw that I wasn't as fast as the others, so he moved me to the slower line where the biggest birds, called "roasters," were shackled. Even more so than on the faster line, the conveyor belt on the "roaster" line consistently clogged with chickens piled on top of each other, often three birds deep.

It was on this line that I saw workers shackle some chickens with their heads caught between their legs and the shackle. Since they weren't hanging upside down, the birds' necks would completely miss the slicing blade, so they may have gone into the scalding tanks while fully conscious. These tanks, true to their name, were filled with scalding-hot water designed to loosen the birds' feathers. Birds who wound up in these tanks endured an even more agonizing and sordid death than those whose necks were slit: they drowned in the hot, feces-choked water.

During one break, I walked outside to check out the trucks waiting to dump the chickens onto the conveyor belt. The chickens were literally packed wing to wing and the crates were so small that the birds couldn't even stand up. Scattered throughout the trucking area were dying birds who had fallen off the truck during the unloading process. These birds were clearly injured, but none of the workers paid any attention to them. No efforts were made to end their suffering, and they were left to die, presumably from dehydration or their injuries.

During one lunch, I went back into the hanging room while my co-workers ate lunch in the cafeteria.

The belt was close to overloaded with birds. Many were injured and dying, and others were already dead. Chickens were lying on top of each other so the ones at the bottom of the piles had to struggle against the weight of so many others just to stick their heads up to breathe.

While I've worked for humane organizations for roughly a decade, the weeks I spent undercover at the slaughter plant taught me many lasting lessons. Perhaps the most important was that while disregard for even the most basic interests of animals is commonplace across industries, the most pressing cruelty concern is the inherent, systematic abuses that millions of birds endure at poultry slaughterhouses all over the country.

Even if every worker handled the animals with the utmost care—which would be impossible, because of the speed of the kill lines—the birds would still suffer dramatically because of the unnaturally rapid growth that increases the chance of skeletal and muscular problems; the transport from the factory farms to the slaughterhouse where they're packed into small cages; the dumping of them on a conveyor belt from their transport trucks; the shackling of their legs into metal restraints; the slicing of their necks while they're fully conscious; and the drowning in scalding tanks for those birds who don't have their throats cut.

It's shameful that while we take so much from these animals, we can't even afford them a less-cruel death. Chickens have the same spark of life as our pets at home. They have the same desire to avoid suffering and to follow their nature. Yet, we treat chickens so cruelly that similar abuses inflicted upon dogs or cats would warrant criminal charges.

Nathan Runkle from the nonprofit Mercy for Animals shared this story with me, from one of his undercover investigators.

Undercover at an Egg Farm

In January and February of 2008, I worked at one of California's largest egg farms—which are a series of massive, enclosed metal buildings. They are all hidden by crops planted around them, their position given away only by the stench of tons of manure and biosecurity signs posted nearby.

The buildings themselves were either one or two stories tall, the larger ones designed to have manure piled up in the first floor with the birds housed up above. Ventilation fans covered the walls; white feathers plastered to their casings and dust formed from excrement caking their blades. The first time I stepped inside one of these sheds, the scene was an assault on the senses and my eyes immediately began to water. An incomprehensible number of lives were crammed inside wire cages four rows high and so far into the distance I couldn't see them through the dust-filled air. Taking in a single breath threatened to choke me, and I had to fight not to go into a coughing fit without a dust mask on. Walking near the cages, the birds inside began making shrieking calls so loud I had to yell to co-workers standing right next to me to be heard. Hens were packed wing to wing and chest to tail in the cages. Not one could spread her wings fully, and they constantly rubbed up against each other and the cage wire to turn around or move toward their feed troughs.

I realized that on industrial egg farms, hens are viewed and treated as commodities. None of these hens is given a name. None of these hens is even given a number. Although each of their lives has a beginning and an end, their individual stories are hard to tell to those who haven't been inside these factory farms. In factory egg production, the hens are treated as egg-producing machines.

Hens were kept in the barns for two years, after which time it was determined they were no longer "productive" enough for the company. For older hens, the broken remnants of their wing feathers lay over pink skin covered in small scratches that were scabbed over or openly bleeding. Many hens had infected wounds on their faces and eyes, had prolapsed uteruses, or had become so sick and lethargic they simply lay at the fronts of the cages breathing in shallow gasps while their cage mates trampled them. Many of these dying hens were cold to the touch and unresponsive to my handling them.

Workers were responsible for pulling dead hens out of the barns every day, and would pull out hens who were crippled and blocking eggs from rolling out of the cages. The workers were supposed to kill the hens by breaking their necks, in either of two methods. The more common method was pulling the hens' necks until the vertebrae separated. A worker demonstrated the technique by pulling a hen's head while he held her body under one armpit. She flapped her wings and kicked her legs frantically. He then held her neck out to me so I could feel the spinal cord where the two vertebrae were pulled apart. I had no way of knowing whether this method had actually cut the spinal cord, and the hens would always flop around on the ground for a minute or two after it was done. A less common method was to swing a hen by her head so that her vertebrae broke and cut the spinal cord. This was done less often, since the birds would release their bowels when it was done, and feces would go flying around in a circle as they were spun.

At one egg site, a worker would not kill the crippled birds he pulled out of cages; instead, he would leave them on the floor, unable to move, to be collected later. I found some inside the trash cans used to collect dead chickens—live, breathing birds buried underneath the dead.

Bird injuries and neglect were common at the farm. I remember coming across one bird that had a wound I can only describe as a crater in her side. I found her lying in her cage, missing most of her feathers on her exposed right side. She didn't move as I lifted her through the cage door, examining a wound about three inches across her torso. It was sunken in at the center and built up around the edges, openly bleeding in several areas. I set her on the floor, where she lay without opening her eyes or lifting her head. She was like many hens I found, their faces and heads pressed painfully against moving egg conveyor belts from sliding partially under their cages' front walls. Drool oozed out of their beaks and their bodies didn't even twitch as they were slowly mutilated by the claws of other hens who were standing over the trapped birds without anywhere else to go inside these tiny enclosures. She counted as nothing now, being unable to consume feed and therefore unable to produce eggs.

I wondered how long she had endured her current state, and how much pain it took to keep her from opening her eyes or calling out. I imagined she was dehydrated and starving from being unable to stand and get food or water, but figured that was a minor discomfort compared to the pain of an infected, open wound that crippled her. I wanted to help her; I wanted to take her from the farm and try to have her healed. That would not be possible, I knew.

Many cages became damaged over time, their floorings rusting out and breaking apart. Frequently, birds in bottom-level cages had to deal with another problem: dead hens left to rot on their floorings beneath their feet. Bottom-level cages were so dark it was impossible to see inside them without a flashlight, and workers responsible for pulling dead hens from cages frequently missed corpses on the bottom row. Eventually, the dead bodies would become trampled to a flat-tened mass, covering much of the cage wire. Feces would then pile up on the bodies, further coating the floorings. Eggs laid by hens would then end up stuck inside the cages instead of rolling under the cages' front walls to the collection belts, and would eventually break and rot.

After two years, when the hens were no longer productive enough, they were killed through a process called depopulation. Workers would move through the aisles with metal carts with carbon dioxide canisters attached to them, filling the carts with hens by shoving them through metal lids on the carts' tops and sides. The workers moved at a rapid pace, grabbing two hens at once. Pulling them out of cages by their necks, wings, or legs with enough force to break their bones, the workers twisted and yanked the birds from the enclosures. If chickens were caught on each other or the cage wire, the workers pulled as hard as they could to tear them free, leaving legs ripped from the hens' bodies behind in the cage floorings. Everywhere near the workers, hens were flapping their wings into each other and the cage wire, frantically calling out and running into the cage walls in a futile attempt to escape the imminent, certainly terrifying, danger. When the workers put the hens into the carts, they slammed the birds down as hard as they could, the hens screaming as they broke through the cart doors and into the poison chamber. Occasionally, a hen would come hopping back out of the doorway, crying out and flapping her wings as quickly as she could, struggling to slip under the battery cages to escape into the manure pit below. Once in the manure pit, her slow death from her injuries or from lack of food or water was sure to follow.

After giving two years of their lives to produce eggs for the company, the hens were rewarded with a brutal death. Sent off to a rendering plant and then combined with cornmeal, the hens' bodies became an ingredient for chicken feed.

And this is what happens to dairy cows . . .

In December 2008, I was hired as a maintenance worker at a large dairy farm. During the six weeks I worked there, I witnessed animal abuse on a massive scale. Although there were many instances of sadistic workers hitting cows for fun, or unnecessarily using electric prods, most abuse was institutional in nature, done not for pleasure but for profit. On this mega dairy farm, over 7,000 cows live in overcrowded, highly unsanitary conditions. They are mutilated, drugged, neglected, left to endure a variety of painful illnesses, and emotionally traumatized by forced separation from their young. The realities of industrial dairy farming are a well-kept secret, nothing like the idyllic dairy farms seen on milk cartons and television ads. During the course of my employment, I encountered thousands of animals that bore the cost of this deception. These are a few of their stories.

It's my second day on the job, and I'm repairing a broken gate in the birthing area, a remote corner of a huge barn where expecting cows are brought to deliver their young. Number 70426, a four-year-old Holstein cow, has just begun to give birth. A worker arrives carrying an archaic-looking metal device that he clamps between the mother cow's nostrils, tethering her in place. He then walks behind her and wraps a steel chain around the emerging forelegs of the birthing calf, putting all of his weight into yanking it out.

The calf falls to the ground with a thud and lies startled on the barren concrete floor. She has a distinctive look, all white except for prominent black markings around her eyes and another at the base of her tail. Her wide, doe-eyes survey her surroundings for the first time before settling on her mom.

Once the worker releases 70426, she makes a beeline directly to her newborn calf, contentedly comforting her with gentle licks. This heartwarming scene is interrupted after only mere minutes, when the worker returns, abruptly grabs the calf and begins to drag her away by one hind leg.

Number 70426 runs behind her calf as they each bellow in distress. When the calf is dragged behind a locked gate, her mother presses her body against the gate and cries out, filling the barn with a sound reminiscent of a tornado siren. But the gate doesn't budge. This is the last time she will ever see her calf, and I feel like she realizes it.

Numbr 70426 continues to call for her baby throughout the afternoon. When she notices me watching, she begins alternating her attention between the gate and me, bellowing with increased urgency. I have to wonder if she is just afraid, or if she is actually pleading for my help. I know that she goes through this every year, but by the looks of her, it never gets easier.

Most calves born on this farm are unwanted by the industry and sent to slaughter when they are only a few days old; however, some females are raised to take their mothers' places. 70426's calf, issued the number 21562, is about to begin a life of intensive milk production.

When she is only weeks old, 21562's horns and tail are amputated. No anesthesia is used. I watch as she is muzzled and tied to a post with the same halter rope used on her mother a month earlier. Using a hot iron scoop, a barn worker begins a process called "disbudding," literally digging the formative horn buds out of her skull. I'll never forget the sight of the smoke billowing from the calf's head as the hot iron met her skin, coupled with the sizzling sound and smell of seared tissue.

"It's incredibly f***ing painful," is how my supervisor explains the process to me. As the worker burns into her skull with the device, 21562 attempts to buck, cries out and tries to escape, but in her ad hoc restraints, she can only produce a muffled moan, before she begins to shake, and finally, collapses.

Unfazed, the worker grabs her tail, yanks her back up, and callously digs his thumb and forefinger into her eye sockets, painfully restricting her motion even further, as he resumes his work.

When the horns are fully burned away, she is then "tail docked." The worker uses a steel clamp to remove a portion of 21562's tail, slicing through her skin, bone, and nerve endings as she kicks and continues to bellow in distress. When she is finally released from the muzzle, saliva pours from her mouth.

Disbudding is an almost universal mutilation carried out on calves raised in intensive confinement on dairy factory farms. When she matures, 21562 will spend every day in a crowded indoor pen, backed up against hundreds of other cows, each vying for space in this narrow, concrete enclosure. The pens are never properly cleaned, forcing her to live in her own bacteria-laden manure. She will only leave this space when she is herded to the milking parlor, milked for five minutes by an automated machine, and returned to her pen. Unlike the pastoral images stamped on the products in which her milk will be sold, 21562 will never graze outside, and will be deprived of access to sunshine, open space, fresh air, and a normal diet.

Cows at this facility are expected to produce upwards of 80 pounds of milk each day—more than five times what they produce naturally. Milk production is bolstered by a foreign diet of grain, longer hours of artificial light, and the routine use of antibiotics, steroids, and the controversial growth hormone rBST. Above all, her milk production is manipulated through repeated impregnation.

My supervisor explained that when a cow begins to produce less than 65 pounds of milk a day, she is "freshened," meaning artificially inseminated to restimulate lactation, typically as soon as two months after her most recent calving. Such an intensive breeding regimen coupled with overmilking is known to cause malnutrition, mastitis (a painful udder inflammation that increases pus levels in milk), abomasal displacement (stomach distention), leg spraddling (crippling), and uterine prolapses (inversion of the uterus, which reduces blood flow and causes decay). Each of these painful afflictions was common at this facility.

Number 46570 endured a lifetime under these conditions before succumbing to a crippling joint infection. She developed a bad sore where her back leg repeatedly chafed on her concrete "bed." The open wound became impacted with manure until it swelled to the size of a softball, visibly dripping pus from a deep abscess in the center. When her condition had fully deteriorated, she was brought to a section of the farm designated for "downers," cows too sick or injured to support their own weight.

I checked on 46570 a week later and was dismayed, if not surprised, to learn that she still hadn't received any meaningful veterinary care. Her cloudy eyes were flared open with an intense look I had seen many times before—an expression of unimaginable suffering. Her right foreleg spasmed involuntarily, and as she breathed in short, heavy bursts, I could hear the crunching noise of her grinding jaw.

Another week went by and she still lay in the same place. By now, she had become extremely thin, far too weak to even lift her head to drink. I sought out the facility's only veterinarian, who insisted that she might still get up if given time.

Although this rationalization was beyond unlikely—downed cows almost never get up after three days—there may have been another reason for prolonging her suffering. Recent legislation banned the sale of downers for human consumption, but not for use in animal by-products. I learned that this loophole means there's a the financial incentive for dairy facilities to withhold humane euthanasia until a downer can be sold to a rendering facility, which will process her into the raw ingredients of products like soap and dog food.

Respite finally came during the third week, and sure enough, it was in the form of a rendering truck. She lay motionless as a chain was strapped around her leg and she was dragged into the cargo hold.

My eyes followed her until they settled on the nursery pen where I first saw 70426's emotional separation from her last calf, 21562. It was a cynical reminder that this cycle of life, death, pain, and profit would continue, not just on this factory farm, but on thousands across the nation.

My experiences indicate that, despite the industry's claims, there is little for the modern dairy cow to be "happy" about. These gentle, intelligent creatures

are overdriven from the day they are born, and aban-
doned as soon as they begin to wear out. If the industry thought these practices were defensible, they
would not be so committed to concealing the truth.

These are not isolated incidents. I know you want to believe
that they are, but they aren't. Every time an investigator goes
undercover, these sorts of routine horrors and abuses come
to light. Every time.

Hard as it is to face, when we know the truth of what's going on, we can choose freely and wisely what to eat. Some will
say, "But what about 'humanely raised' meat?" or "Aren't the
ranchers who grow organic, grass-fed beef and poultry and
pork doing things differently?" Yes, a little. For that tiny percentage of "humanely raised" animals—the "lucky ones"
who are given room to turn around, lie down, or stretch their
wings—life may indeed be a tad bit better, but it is far from
"good." Even the animals who are raised on smaller farms
(minuscule number though that is) are ultimately sent—
often by a long and harrowing truck drive in all kinds of severe weather—to the very same horrid slaughterhouses that
kill their factory-farmed kin.

I recently saw a video shot by a University of Texas film
student called *Free Range?* The student, Neel Parekh, was
allowed to shoot openly on a free-range farm. You see their
chickens being slaughtered in a manner identical to that of
factory-farmed chickens, and they are clearly still conscious when they are immersed—necks sliced open and
blood pouring out—in scalding hot water for feather re-
moval. Anyone who is thinking about "humane meat":

please do an online search for, and watch, this young man's video.

And remember this: the vast majority—more than 95 percent—of animals people eat are raised in factory farms and not on the old-fashioned family farms of memory.

When you eat a plant-based diet, you make a powerful promise to yourself: you say no to causing needless suffering; you say no to hurting animals.

PROMISE 9:

You Will Be Following the Wisdom of the Great Spiritual Traditions

Did you know?

- Saint Francis of Assisi ate a largely vegetarian diet and John Wesley (founder of the Methodist Church) was a strict vegetarian.
- The diet God ordains in Eden is strictly vegetarian (Genesis 1:29–30). A long line of Jewish and Christian commentators have taught that granting permission to eat meat is portrayed in the Bible as a concession to human weakness.
- In Buddhism, Jainism, and Hinduism, vegetarianism is a part of daily life.
- Indian traditions teach that vegetarian diets modify the chemistry and hormonal balance of our bodies, promoting calm, focus, and increased energy.

- The Prophet Muhammad had compassion for dogs and preached compassion for all animals.
- Today in the U.S., kosher and halal meats are not slaughtered any more humanely than any other meats.
- Many spiritual practices view vegetarianism as a basic prerequisite, opening human possibilities that are closed to those who cannot curb the desire for flesh.

When I began considering my diet as a way to practice my spiritual beliefs, I came up against so much inner turmoil. How could eating meat, dairy, and eggs be wrong when so many people do it daily and with gusto? If long-standing faith traditions hold that eating animals is acceptable, who was I to question those traditions?

And yet, especially after watching behind-the-scenes video of what happens to animals as they become our food, I remained troubled, on a spiritual level, at the thought of eating them. If I am someone who wants peace in the world, how can I make peace with my part in the system of institutionalized cruelty and misery toward animals? How could I feel peaceful inside if I continued to collude with this bringing of suffering? The more I meditated on it, the clearer it became: Choosing to be a veganist is not just about my physical health, it is about the well-being of all creatures of this planet; it is a vital part of an awake and aware spiritual practice as well. It's not just that I choose not to contribute to the suffering of animals; my vegan choices also allow me to become the person I want to be.

Investigating the Great Faith Traditions

For a long time I had the idea that the great faith traditions aren't concerned with food or even with our relationship to animals, but as I gave it serious thought, that didn't seem correct to me. How could any wisdom tradition that has endured for many hundreds or thousands of years not have reflected on so fundamental a question as how we relate to these fellow creatures? Animals are so totally in our power, after all, and isn't spirituality in part a matter of how we choose to treat the powerless?

I decided to do some searching—both soul searching and researching the world's spiritual traditions—to find out what they really suggest about the question of eating animals.

The first thing that became clear was that virtually all spiritual traditions have indeed considered the question of whether it is ethical for humans to eat animals. My initial explorations only skimmed the surface, but even so it was easy to see that spiritual leaders throughout the ages have grappled with the contradictions inherent in following and advocating a peaceful, humane existence while killing and eating animals. For Christians and Jews the dilemma is so central that it is addressed in the very first chapter of the first book of the Bible, Genesis, preceding even the Ten Commandments! The first thing God does after creating humans is call humanity to steward the earth and its creatures, but the second thing God does is declare, "See, I have given you every plant-yielding seed that is upon the face of all the earth, and every tree with seed in its fruit; you shall have them for food" (Genesis 1:29–30). A clear call for vegetarianism, it would seem.

I already knew that important contemporary religious leaders from Pope Benedict XVI to His Holiness the 14th

Dalai Lama had condemned factory farming. What I didn't expect was that it wasn't just a few great lights or just a few religious traditions speaking about meat as a problem. Spiritual traditions have always wrestled with the questions raised by eating animals.

"One of the most striking things one discovers in comparative religion," the historian of religions and Jewish studies scholar Aaron Gross, PhD, explained to me:

> The potential moral danger of meat eating is a major theme across religious traditions. Eating meat is often condemned and, if not, it is surrounded by cautions and restrictions as is the case in Christianity, Islam, and Judaism. Mircea Eliade, arguably the most influential scholar of religion in the twentieth century, in fact argued that the ancient hunter's sympathy for the animals he killed was one of the origins of religion itself. Religion begins in part, Eliade theorized, out of concern about the problem posed by killing in order to live.

It seems that my discomfort with the business of eating meat has ample precedent! So not surprisingly, as soon as I looked, I found numerous spiritual leaders from multiple traditions calling upon us to eat more spiritually and mindfully.

Christian Traditions

A new generation of Christian theologians has shown that the question of food, especially meat, has been one of the great religious questions in Christian history. David Grumett, PhD, and Rachel Muers, PhD, are the first scholars to systematically study the issue. "Nowadays people might think of religion as being about abstract beliefs," explains Grumett, "but if you look back through history it's been very much about people's day-to-day lives, such as what they ate."

Today Christian theologians are rediscovering the links between our dietary and spiritual choices. Many are arguing that vegetarianism is the diet most compatible with Christian values like mercy and compassion. The Anglican priest and Oxford professor Andrew Linzey, PhD, argues that "to stand with Jesus is to . . . honor life for the sake of the Lord of life. . . . To stand for Jesus is to stand for active compassion for the weak, against the principle that might is right." For Linzey, this means Christians should be vegetarian.

Theologians like Linzey, I learned, are part of a long tradition of meat abstainers that stretches back to the origins of Christian faith. The Desert Fathers, fourth-century Christian saints, abstained from meat. The fifteen-hundred-year-old Rule of Saint Benedict, a pillar of monastic spiritual practice, severely restricts meat eating. Under the influence of this rule many contemporary monastic orders, especially in Eastern Christianity, are vegetarian to this day.

Some later Christian leaders were semi-vegetarians, like Saint Francis of Assisi (1182–1226), who avoided meat as best they could. Others, like the founder of Methodism, John Wesley (1703–1791), were full-time vegetarians. Many more were vegetarian for limited periods. Still today there is a vibrant Catholic tradition of giving up some or all meat for Lent, the period before Easter.

While contemporary Christian vegetarianism is usually rooted in ethical concerns about the abuse of creation, historically Christians who chose not to eat flesh also saw their diet as a path to greater spirituality and increased sanctity. Both seem like good reasons to me!

I was delighted to learn about this rich tradition of incorporating vegetarian diets into spiritual practice, but I admit that it surprised me at first. It certainly is not something most Christians in America know about. If you do some searching, though—even simply by searching "Christianity and vegetarianism" on the Internet—it's easy to see just how important the idea of peace among all creatures has been in the Christian moral imagination. Indeed, you don't need to look any farther than the first thirty lines of the Bible: the diet God ordains in Eden is strictly vegetarian! You don't need to take my word for that. Jewish and Christian biblical interpreters have agreed for millennia that Genesis 1:29–30, the verse I quoted at the beginning of this chapter, is proof that humanity's first diet was meat free.

It's a stunning vision when you pause to think about it. When God imagined the perfect world, it was a world where humans did not eat animals, but instead lived on the gifts of food growing on trees and in the ground. According to the biblical narrative, it was only after the fall that humans started eating animals. The ideal is to strive to return to the original perfection. This is why when the prophet Isaiah is describing the messianic era in which the world is again made perfect, he declares that "[t]he wolf shall live with the lamb . . . and the lion shall eat straw like the ox" (Isaiah 11:6–7). Given this, it makes perfect sense that today more Christians are questioning the rightness of eating meat and are turning toward vegetarianism.

The endorsement of vegetarianism in the first chapter of

Genesis is sometimes ignored by Christians who like to emphasize that by the ninth chapter, human beings have been given permission to eat meat. So I decided to look into how that "permission" to eat animals is portrayed in the Bible.

One thing all commentators seem to agree on is that the late tolerance of meat eating doesn't mean that God just "made a mistake" and realized that slaughterhouses were actually a good idea. A long history of Jewish and Christian commentators have taught that granting permission to eat meat is portrayed in the Bible as a concession to human weakness. In the very same biblical verses where permission to eat meat is given, all humanity is required to drain blood, an ancient symbol of life, from the animals. At first draining the blood from animals—still practiced in virtually all slaughterhouses today—just seemed bizarre to me, but scholars have deciphered its meaning: namely, to remind human beings that meat eating was not part of God's original plan.

In an exhaustive 3,000-plus-page analysis of Leviticus, Rabbi Jacob Milgrom, PhD, the foremost biblical expert on this issue, shows that if we want to understand the immense importance the Bible gives to the blood prohibition, we have to look back to the beginning of Genesis. "Above all," Milgrom writes, "it must be recalled that . . . man was initially meant to be a vegetarian. Later, God concedes to man's carnivorous desires: his craving for meat is to be indulged, but he is to abstain from consuming the blood." Milgrom explains that the Bible shows an "uneasiness regarding man's uncontrolled power over animal life. . . . [I]t seeks to curb that power. All men must eschew the lifeblood of the animal by draining it. . . . Mankind has a right to nourishment, not to life. Hence the blood, the symbol of life, must be drained, returned to the universe, to God."

If that seems surprising, it's because of how alienated we are from these issues today. As Milgrom observes, this kind of concern about killing was once much more common: "Anthropological and comparative evidence indicates that the reluctance to kill an animal harks back to a much earlier period." In the end, Milgrom concludes that the blood prohibition is part of a biblical ethic that demands "reverence for life."

Rather than giving humans carte blanche to eat meat, the Bible saddles the practice with restrictions. And if eating meat even from animals raised back in the good old days before intensive confinement and antibiotics and industrial slaughterhouses wasn't endorsed, then what does that suggest about our own day, when animals suffer miserable lives on factory farms and painful deaths in industrial slaughterhouses?

In sum: What would Jesus think of a factory farm? It's one thing to concede that meat eating was temporarily tolerable to ancient herders, but when all you have to do is order something different from a menu or reach for a different part of the supermarket shelf, wouldn't the Christian thing be to choose the more peaceful option?

My Own Spiritual Path

I suppose I should say a bit about my spiritual path: I was baptized a Catholic and thought of myself exclusively as a Christian for many years. Even though today I also find spiritual sustenance from other traditions, my spiritual journey has never led me to reject anything Jesus taught. Everything the churches I attended taught about the life of Jesus—his love for creation, mercy, compassion, and special concern for the powerless—leads me to think he would never have accepted a diet that contributed to the groans of creation. As the Apostle Paul explains in a beautiful passage, it is not only humans that look forward to salvation: "The whole creation has been groaning in labor pains until now" (Romans 8:22). Animals and all the earth are included in God's plan.

I also love that in his first letter to the Thessalonians, Paul calls on the community to "pray ceaselessly." I don't think he meant that we should constantly have our heads bowed, murmuring prayers, but rather that we should live as if we were constantly trying to be the people we are guided to be. Since eating is so central to our lives, it seems to me that eating consciously can be the foundation of our conscious life. It can be our way of praying ceaselessly.

I don't see how the ultimate Good Shepherd, the Prince of Peace, could be okay with a lifestyle that promotes misery and destroys health. Maybe Jesus wasn't a strict vegetarian 2,000 years ago, but there sure is something to the idea that he would be today.

Consider the reflections of the Jesuit priest John Dear, who explains that "today Jesus . . . would want us to change every aspect of our lives, to seek complete physical, spiritual, emotional, and ethical wholeness. . . . So, when we sit down to eat . . . we should also choose to adhere to his life of compassion and nonviolence by maintaining a vegetarian diet." Like Christians have for centuries, he sees a plant-based diet contributing to our spiritual wellness. He adds that "we know that as we practice mercy to one another and to all

God's creatures, we too shall receive mercy and blessings, as Jesus promised in the Beatitudes."

The influential "ecotheologian" Thomas Berry reaches the same conclusion. "Vegetarianism is a way of life that we should all move toward for economic survival, physical well-being, and spiritual integrity." In perhaps his most famous teaching, Berry speaks against the idea that the world is a mere "collection of objects" and insists we look at creation as a "communion of subjects." By leaving animal products out of our diet we welcome into our lives new, more beautiful, and more inspiring ways of being a part of the natural world.

Linzey, Dear, and Berry are speaking for many other Christians past and present who also have found a link between the spiritual life and a life of compassion for animals. The Christian teaching of compassion for animals was especially emphasized by Francis of Assisi. Saint Francis not only spoke eloquently about compassion for animals but also (like Linzey, Dear, and Berry) taught that kindness to animals is good spiritually and promotes peace among humans. "Not to hurt our humble brethren, the animals, is our first duty to them, but to stop there is not enough. We have a higher mission: to be of service to them whenever they require it. If you have people who will exclude any of God's creatures from the shelter of compassion and pity you will have people who will deal likewise with other people."

It feels like this is what was meant when God said we have "dominion" over animals. Rather than exploiting them and using them for our every whim, perhaps we are to take care of them, or at least not to hurt them. In other words, kindness to animals whether expressed in diet or other ways is an essential part of one's spiritual life. This has become my experience in very concrete ways.

For example, after learning the truth about how animals suffer on today's industrialized "farms," I faced a kind of spiritual choice. I could press the facts from my mind and pretend that the violence I was supporting by eating animal products was someone else's responsibility. Had I made that choice it would have shaped the person I am today and my spiritual life in important (and unfortunate) ways. Instead, I listened to my better instincts, and I've found that when you learn to do that with the foods you choose, you learn to do it in many other parts of your life as well. One good deed leads to another.

My friend the novelist Jonathan Safran Foer, who was inspired to commit to vegetarianism by the birth of his first child and wrote a wonderful book about it called *Eating Animals*, put it this way: "Compassion is a muscle that gets stronger with use, and the regular exercise of choosing kindness over cruelty . . . change[s] us." Aligning my diet with my beliefs has helped me become more like the person I want to be.

It's not surprising, really, that when the world's single most influential spiritual leader, Pope Benedict XVI, was asked to comment on the factory farming of animals, he began by saying, "That is a very serious question." If the rest of his answer weren't so insightful, I would be tempted to stop there. It's such an important point: what we choose to eat is "a very serious question." Yet, many of us never ask it. The pope continues, "Animals, too, are God's creatures. . . . Certainly, a sort of industrial use of creatures, so that geese are fed in such a way as to produce as large a liver as possible, or hens live so packed together that they become just caricatures of birds, this degrading of living creatures to a commodity seems to me in fact to contradict the relationship of mutuality that comes across in the Bible." Yes, such practices are indeed degrading to living creatures, but they also degrade our own humanity. Who are we if we not only allow this to happen, but if we purchase the end results of such a miserable process?

Jewish Traditions

What the pope calls a "relationship of mutuality" between humans and animals sounds to my ears similar to the ideal relationship with animals I found expressed in Judaism's rabbinic tradition. Rabbi Moses Maimonides, also simply called Maimonides (1135–1204), was the greatest Jewish scholar of his time. It is said of him that "from Moses to Moses there has been no one like Moses." In Maimonides' most important work, a spiritual guidebook he entitled *The Guide for the Perplexed*, he spends considerable time on the virtue of compassion for animals. Explaining the reason for biblical laws that require a person to show sensitivity to the bonds between mother hens and their chicks, Maimonides explains that there is "no difference . . . between humanity and the other animals" in relation to the pain a mother experiences if she sees her young harmed. "For the love and the tenderness of a mother for her child is not consequent upon reason but upon the activity of the imaginative faculty, which is found in most animals just as it is found in humanity."

Maimonides is not just speaking his own mind here, but

representing an ancient and contemporary practice of compassion for animals that the Jewish tradition has known as *tzaar baalei chayim*. Traditionally *tzaar baalei chayim* has not been interpreted as absolutely requiring vegetarianism, but in the age of factory farming numerous rabbis are going vegetarian and citing this venerable principle. One such rabbi is David Wolpe, the senior rabbi at one of the largest synagogues in the world, Temple Sinai in Los Angeles, who was recently celebrated by *Newsweek* as the "number one pulpit rabbi in America."

Rabbi Wolpe has emphasized that the spiritual benefits of vegetarianism and compassion for animals don't just apply to nonhuman animals. Consider Rabbi Wolpe's discussion of the passage from Maimonides just cited above:

> There is a Jewish law that you're not allowed to take the eggs from a nest without shooing the mother bird away. First you have to get rid of the mother bird so that she won't see you collecting the eggs from the nest. It's a law that's explicit in the Torah. And there are two interpretations of that law. One interpretation following Maimonides is that it is because the bird itself has feelings and you don't want it to see you taking the egg. The other interpretation following Nachmanides is that you shouldn't be so coarse, so insensitive, so cruel, as right in front of a mother to take its young. Both of those interpretations are at play here. It's not only that we shouldn't inflict this kind of pain on animals; it's that we shouldn't be the kind of people who would do it.

I love this idea. Veganism doesn't just mean we are kinder to animals; it allows us to be more like the kind of people that spiritual traditions have always encouraged us to be.

The rabbis I spoke with explained that today many Jews are vegetarian out of concern for animal welfare, but *also* simply as a way to participate in an ancient Jewish practice meant to transform eating into a spiritual activity, the kosher diet. As it turns out virtually all the kosher laws deal with regulating animal products—for example prohibitions against eating pigs or shellfish, or the laws of Jewish religious slaughter.

It's very easy for a vegetarian to keep kosher and even easier for vegans.

Veganism doesn't just mean we are kinder to animals, it allows us to be more like the kind of people that spiritual traditions have always encouraged us to be.

For millennia, Jewish sages have found a teaching in this: the practice of eating kosher is not simply a concession on the vegetarian ideal. A kosher diet is meant to gently lead people back to vegetarianism—back to Eden.

This is where the question, "Well, kosher is at least humane, isn't it?" comes up. To answer this, I spoke with a couple of people who have firsthand experience in today's kosher slaughterhouses. One of the most knowledgeable was Philip Schein. This is his story in his own words.

Philip Schein's Story:
The Question of Kosher Meat

I am a cruelty investigator for the world's largest animal protection group, People for the Ethical Treatment of Animals, or PETA. It's a life I never could have imagined. I grew up eating meat, not protesting it. I am Jewish and I was always told that kosher meat was humane. I was told that how we treated those beings in our power mattered greatly, that it was what defined us as human beings. It was a way of approaching daily life that made me proud to be Jewish.

Today I have conducted more than ten undercover investigations at major kosher slaughter facilities from Nebraska to Uruguay. This firsthand experience on kill floors quickly shattered any naïve hopes I held out that kosher meant humane.

In South America, which supplies a large percentage of kosher beef to Israel and the United States, the standard method of kosher slaughter is the "shackle and hoist" technique, in which cattle are chained, tripped, and restrained on the ground while their throats are cut, and then they are hoisted immediately into the air to be bled out while still conscious and struggling. In the U.S., at what was at the time the world's single largest kosher slaughter facility, I've seen workers systematically hacking out the tracheas and esophagi of conscious and wide-eyed cattle. I've seen workers shock animals in the face with electric prods and let animals languish for minutes as the result of sloppy religious slaughter techniques. All these violations are a matter of public record now and they were widely reported on in the media. You can see the videos at www.humanekosher.com. These practices are not standard and certainly not required by kosher law, but I'm ashamed how many other examples I could give of egregious cruelty at kosher facilities. And even more shameful than any of these abuses is the response to them by kosher certification authorities.

I expected these violations of the Jewish principle of compassion to animals to be condemned. I also expected that the meat from these slaughterhouses would be declared unkosher, but that is not what happened. Many in the Jewish community protested, but the leadership of the kosher industry insisted and still insists that the flesh of animals who die torturous deaths—even animals dismembered while conscious—can be perfectly kosher. It's not that the situation is necessarily worse in kosher slaughterhouses than in conventional slaughter facilities—the problems with cruelty at mainstream slaughterhouses are arguably worse overall. But I expected kosher production to reflect a higher ethical standard. Sadly, what I witnessed in both kosher and nonkosher facilities is that suffering and cruelty is systemic in all forms of industrialized slaughter.

And regardless of what happens at the slaughterhouse, almost all the animals killed for kosher meat are supplied by the very same cruel factory farms that supply animals for conventional slaughter.

If kosher was once supposed to be an honorable compromise with the vegetarian ideal depicted in Genesis, it's long ceased to be. I'm still proud of Jewish dietary traditions, but today it's the growing movement of Jewish vegetarianism that I find inspiring. I'm not against kosher, but I am against what passes as kosher today. As the Nobel Laureate and Yiddish writer I. B. Singer put it, "I'm not against organized religion, but I don't take part in it . . . when they interpret their religious books as being in favor of meat-eating. . . . [Vegetarianism] is my protest against the conduct of the world. To be a vegetarian is to disagree—to disagree with the course of things today . . . starvation, cruelty—we must make a statement against these things. Vegetarianism is my statement. And I think it's a strong one."

The Jewish leaders I've researched unanimously agree that the ideal of kosher slaughter is to create a quick and painless death—something the laws of kosher share with the Muslim dietary laws, called Halal. They also agreed with Philip that the reality today is far different.

Muslim Teachings

The same unfortunate situation also exists in the production of Halal meat, even though Muslim tradition too has teachings exhorting its followers to compassion for animals. One tenth-century Iraqi religious tale even imagines the animals of the world issuing a lawsuit against humanity before the divine court because of humanity's disregard for the natural

world (an Islamic case for animal rights?). The animals explain that before the creation of Adam, "we were fully occupied in caring for our broods and rearing our young with all
the good food and water God had allotted us, secure and un-
molested in our own lands. Night and day we praised and
sanctified God, and God alone."

The animals protest that after the creation of human beings, they were treated mercilessly. "Whoever fell into their
hands was . . . slaughtered and flayed. . . . [Humans] ripped
open his belly, cut off his limbs and broke his bones, tore out
his eyes; plucked his feathers or sheared off his hair or fleece,
and put him onto the fire to be cooked, or on the spit to be
roasted, or subjected him to even more dire tortures, whose full
extent is beyond description." It sounds like I'm quoting from
an animal protection pamphlet, but this is a thousand-year-old
Arabic text! Other tales tell of the Prophet Muhammad's compassion for animals and his special affection for dogs.

Much more significant for Muslims, though, is a famous
line in the Koran that beautifully expresses the idea that animals too are "good Muslims" and obey God in their own
fashion. "There is not an animal that lives on the earth, nor
a being that flies on its wings, but forms part of communities
like you. . . . [T]hey all shall be gathered to their Lord in the
end" (6:38). The word for "communities" used in this verse
is the sacred Arabic word *ummah*, which is still today the
common term used by Muslims to refer to *human* religious
communities. Wherever the teachings of Muhammad, Moses,
and Jesus may differ, they clearly agree that God enjoined humans to avoid cruelty to animals. They may not have advocated vegetarianism in their own day, but the real question

is what these spiritual giants would say while standing in the shadow of today's meat, dairy, and egg industries?

Buddhism, Jainism, and Hinduism
While the Abrahamic traditions of Christianity, Islam, and Judaism have championed values that lead one toward vegetarianism, the religious traditions that stem from India, such as Buddhism, Jainism, and Hinduism, have gone much further. In these traditions vegetarianism has not only been the theoretical ideal of the perfect world, but has been advocated as a basic part of the spiritual life. In America we are fortunate today that more restaurants are adding vegetarian sections to their menus, but meat-centered food is still the norm. In India today, the situation is often reversed. Instead of talking about "regular" and vegetarian food like we do here, restaurants are described as "veg or non-veg." Eating animals is the aberrant diet!

The spiritual traditions originating in India, which today have almost 2 billion followers worldwide, have dealt thoughtfully with violence and have taught that killing and consuming animals goes hand in hand with violence to other humans. A guiding principle of all three traditions is ahimsa, literally "nonviolence," the doctrine that all living beings are sacred and that we should avoid injuring them. Many Americans know of ahimsa through the teachings of Mahatma Gandhi, the "father" of modern India and a key inspiration to Dr. Martin Luther King Jr. (King's widow, Coretta Scott King, was vegan until her death, and his son, Dexter King, still is).

The principle of ahimsa exposes the disconnected relationship that many of us have with our food. It is difficult and shocking to look at a piece of meat on your plate and visualize the violence that brought it there. Most of us, if we really thought about it, would find it repellent to personally commit such a violent act when so many nonviolent (and healthier) alternatives exist to nourish us. This kind of reasoning has led countless practitioners of Buddhism, Jainism, Hinduism, and others inspired by these teachings to become lifelong vegetarians.

And ahimsa isn't the only reason given for a vegetarian diet in these traditions. Meditative discipline and traditional Indian medicine, Ayurveda, teach that meat can harm health and reduce life span, something Western science has also confirmed, as we have seen. Indian traditions also teach that vegetarian diets modify the chemistry and hormonal balance of our bodies, promoting calm, focus, and increased energy. For many spiritual practices, vegetarianism is seen as a basic prerequisite, opening human possibilities closed to those who cannot curb the desire for flesh.

The Buddhist scriptures relate that the Enlightened One advised that "those who keep close company with me must not eat meat. Even if, in a gesture of faith, almsgivers provide them with meat, they must shrink from it as they would shrink from the flesh of their own children," because "eating meat destroys the attitude of great compassion."

Thich Nhat Hanh, a world-famous Vietnamese Buddhist monk who has inspired millions of Westerners, strongly advocates becoming vegan or at least significantly reducing the amount of meat you eat. Hanh likes to emphasize just how many wonderful reasons there are to motivate this diet: among other things, he says, it is a way to stand against global warming, land degradation, and water pollution.

Perhaps Thich Nhat Hanh's major teaching is "mindfulness," a practice of deep awareness of how we are living in the world from moment to moment. Hahn encourages mindfulness in all areas of our lives and, since eating is something we do multiple times every day, eating mindfully is especially important. Hahn explains that we don't need any special teaching to realize the spiritual advantages of vegetarianism. All we need to do is eat mindfully.

Hanh teaches that by eating mindfully, for example visualizing for a moment how that meat on your plate *really* got there, will make us realize that by eating meat "we are eating the flesh of our own children."

Hanh doesn't mean that literally of course, but if we think about the impact of the meat we eat, we will realize how we are harming the entire planet and ultimately hurting ourselves, especially the young among us. By our indifference to cruelty and our direct harm to the environment, we create a worse rather than better world for our children. In essence, Hanh is saying that if we listen to our better instincts, they will naturally guide us toward vegetarianism.

Try a thought experiment yourself. Imagine what it takes for a piece of chicken leg to end up on your plate (confinement, transportation to slaughter, slaughtering, defeathering, skinning, butchering, slicing up, and cooking). Now imagine the process involved in eating an apple (pluck it off the tree) or loaf of bread (harvesting the grain, milling it ino flour, baking). Would you rather have your energies contribute to a world of slaughter or one of harvest? It's a decision we make every day.

I came away from my research and soul searching with the clear perception that a shared directive runs through all the major religions and wisdom philosophies, and it is this: cultivate compassion, and do so actively. If we do nothing else but this, our lives will be spiritually successful.

PROMISE 10:

You Will Evolve—and Take the World with You

I'M SO GLAD YOU ARE STILL WITH ME. I HOPE THAT AS YOU HAVE read along you have made some new connections and seen the immense promise and possibility that lies in the choice to become a veganist. I think it is safe to say that whether we are talking about healthy trimming down, living longer and better, reducing animal suffering, helping the global poor, or shrinking your carbon footprint, there are few things you can do that have the broad impact of a plant-based diet. This is why I've spent so much of this book documenting these benefits and telling the stories of those for whom a vegan turn has been transformative.

Perhaps the greatest promise of a plant-based diet, in my view, is that it can help us evolve. A plant-based diet gives all of us an opportunity to be transformative agents in the task of creating a more perfect world. This isn't hyperbole. If our intentions are to have peace, happiness, kindness, and abundance, we have to put those intentions into action. Beyond wanting peace, we have to sow the seeds of peace. There are only so many ways to do this, and each one is of great consequence. It's really amazing when you think about it: each time we eat we are given an opportunity to make the world kinder and to reduce the harm we cause. *And* to benefit our own health and vitality as we do so!

Our food choices affect others like virtually nothing else we do, rippling outward and multiplying their impact day by day, year by year, meal by meal. Every time we choose what to eat we vote in the most important and most democratic election on the planet. And after each breakfast we cook and each lunch we order, the results are calculated and the world is inched in one direction or the other. In 2006, for example, the percentage of the world's population that was clinically obese quietly surpassed the number of people afflicted by hunger, a clear result of the growth of high-meat diets. Talk about ironies.

Every time we choose what to eat we vote in the most important and most democratic election on the planet.

As we've seen, every plant-based meal helps heal this sad situation. Every time we eat we affect what foods our supermarkets carry, what our neighbors eat, and what future generations will eat. Each food choice ripples out into the world and into the future in ways that few if any other daily decisions do. Eating is *the* paradigmatic social act, breaking bread the most elementary gesture of hospitality. One thing you can be sure of is that even if you are the first among your family or friends to lean toward veganism, you won't be the last. You will influence others. Even if you don't talk about it you'll find that people will come to you with questions. You will be a part of helping society reach a higher level of consciousness. A plant-based diet is the promise that keeps on giving.

What's Stopping Us?

In my experience once people learn the facts and hear real-life stories, the old-fashioned idea that animal foods are necessary quickly becomes as persuasive as stories about the tooth fairy. Winning "the argument" for plant-based diets, with your conscience or your neighbor, however, is an important but in the end relatively easy victory. The more challenging part is putting it into practice (much advice on that in the afterword)!

So, what to do about that?

Openness to new ideas is one of the things that I love about Americans—we're always ready to hear about another, better way to do things. And while we have no doubt enjoyed meat with our potatoes for some time, we are above all a practical people, especially when it comes to the food we eat. Even back when Americans first won independence, writes the Texas State University history professor James McWilliams, they made a "concerted turn back toward culinary simplicity." Whereas in Europe eating was often an elaborate affair, Americans worked "under the assumption that eating was more of a practical activity . . . than a ceremonial one. Just as American culture had become more pragmatic, so had its food."

Practically speaking, there are too many commonsense advantages of a plant-based diet to ignore. Still, when our hearts and minds open to the promises of a plant-based diet, there is often another part of ourselves that is busy scripting "top ten" lists of reasons why we can't do it. It's human nature to throw up resistance to important change. Despite all the common sense a vegan diet makes, it's easy to feel overwhelmed instead of inspired by its promises. We can know everything there is to know about how changing our diet could lead to personal growth but still falter, at least at first.

Perhaps the greatest promise of a plant-based diet, in my view, is that it can help us evolve. A plant-based diet gives all of us an opportunity to be transformative agents in the task of creating a better world.

Yet, as with other important changes, persistence pays off, and it's by overcoming these internal obstacles and putting the changes that we know are right into practice—perhaps by leaning in to them gradually and at a pace that is comfortable—that we reap the biggest rewards. As we realize our capacity to listen to our better instincts, this powers us on even further. And once we get that momentum going, a quantum leap becomes possible, and we transform not only ourselves but our families, communities, and nations along with us.

What is it that makes that leap possible? And what is it that's stopping us from doing what we know is a good move all around?

Lifting Out of an Addiction

Knowledge itself is pretty inspiring. For many people, just learning about all the benefits of plant-based food is enough to prompt a leap of action. And for most, once they ease animal products from their diet, they quickly experience the personal benefits and their commitment to the diet grows.

As I've emphasized from the beginning of this book, though, for many of us the switch can be much harder (I certainly didn't transition easily or overnight). Knowledge may inspire, but it's not the only ingredient needed to make a substantial and lasting change. Remember Natala's story in Promise 2? "I would sit in my car and cry outside of sub shops, just wanting a tuna melt." Some folks sincerely want to make the change but struggle against their bodies' cravings for animal products. It's important to remember that these cravings *will go away if they are not indulged*. That said, many people find that their knowledge of the benefits of a vegan diet isn't enough to resist a meat or cheese itch.

If you find it's hard to give up meat, dairy, or eggs, there is a good reason for that: medical doctors like Neal Barnard have long talked about how animal products are habit-forming. Giving them up is not as hard as breaking a smoking or alcohol addiction, but it poses many of the same kinds of challenges, especially psychologically. Getting off animal products can involve breaking what medical professionals have begun to call a "food addiction." In speaking with medical students, Dr. Barnard invites them to imagine the following scenario:

> The patient stumbles into the doctor's office. He has a bleary look in his eyes and a bulbous red nose covered

with broken veins. With slurred speech, he tells the doctor about his repeated hospitalizations for cirrhosis of the liver, his gradually worsening mental acuity, and his personal life marked by inability to hold a job and several arrests for abuse of his wife.

The doctor shakes his head with disbelief. How could one man have so many seemingly unrelated problems? Apparently, he has a visual problem, a skin problem, a neurological problem, a liver problem, mild dementia, and recurrent interpersonal difficulties. No doubt he'll need referrals to many different specialists and a lot of medication.

Well, obviously, the situation is absurd. No one would miss the diagnosis of alcoholism. But let's imagine a different case. A man walks into the doctor's office. He complains of constipation that has bothered him since childhood, and he has been steadily gaining weight. His cholesterol level has tended to run high, and a few years ago he developed high blood pressure and borderline diabetes. He has had recurrent episodes of gout, sometimes requiring hospitalization.

To most doctors, these are unrelated diagnoses, and they are treated with an enormous number of drugs. But an increasing number of doctors recognize this symptom cluster as having all the hallmarks of addiction—an addiction to fatty, cholesterol-laden foods.

Can people really be *addicted* to meat or cheese? "An increasing body of evidence," explains Dr. Barnard, "suggests that they may well be." That isn't all bad news. Once we see that we are facing an addiction, the possibility of making a profound shift is opened.

You know you are addicted to a food if despite knowing it is bad for you and despite wanting to change, you still keep eating it. Addiction means that a craving has more control over your behavior than you do. Almost by definition an addiction takes some effort to overcome, but in more than a few ways, those that struggle the most with going vegan are those who benefit the most. Only challenges make us stronger. How we respond to our addiction to animal products is an opportunity. A vegan diet is a meaningful victory that anyone who sets their mind to it can achieve.

If you want to read more on how to break through addiction, there is a whole section on it in my book *Quantum Wellness*. I will tell you one thing, though: whatever your fatal attraction is, at best it keeps you in a holding pattern and at worst it puts you in a downward spiral. In the case of being addicted to certain foods like meat or cheese, that downward spiral can be obesity, disease, or loss of sex drive, energy, or self-esteem. It can also involve a deadening of your awareness and empathy. When you know what the end results of poor food choices are (and you definitely know by now!), you can challenge yourself to break free in much the same way you leave off other addictive substances. The more you get the addictive foods out of your diet, the less you will actually crave them. Consider that when we eat uncontrollably like drug addicts, it is probably because we have grown desensitized to the tastes of healthier foods, and need more and more of fatty, rich junk food for the same rush of pleasure. Nothing—no habit or food or substance—should ever own us, so it's worth gently pushing ourselves into a new way of eating. Just keep leaning in to healthier choices, and soon enough your body will reject the bad stuff. You simply have to get used to good food; give yourself the time to adjust—it will happen.

A Tipping Point with Food?

When we overcome our cravings and let the better side of our nature prevail over this decision about food, we aren't just changing any old habit. Food shapes us inside and out. If we can turn our glimpses of a better way to eat into a new way of eating, then we take a quantum leap forward. What kind of people would we become if we exercised the muscle of awareness and compassion every time we ordered a meal?

We've all noticed that the benefits of a plant-based diet have been discussed more and more prominently in the last decade. Movies from *Food, Inc.* to *Earthlings*, and books from Jonathan Safran Foer's *Eating Animals* to Rory Freedman and Kim Barnouin's *Skinny Bitch* have brought the latest facts about food to new audiences. The U.S. market for vegetarian specialty foods exceeded a billion dollars for the first time shortly after the new millennium and continues to grow. When an activity attracts a critical mass of participants, the point at which its expanding influence is nearly unstoppable, that is known as a tipping point. Diseases, hobbies, fashions, tastes of all kinds have experienced this tipping point phenomenon. Many signs now suggest that as a society we may be about to reach a tipping point in our relationship with food. I have no doubt we are at a threshold.

Consider some of the things that have happened since the beginning of the twenty-first century. Working in association with the Monday Campaigns, the Johns Hopkins Bloomberg School of Public Health has advocated for "Meatless Monday," becoming the first major U.S. public health institution to endorse a program that explicitly sets out to reduce meat consumption. The Meatless Monday initiative pursues the modest goal of a 15 percent reduction in meat intake by encouraging people all over the world to make their Mondays vegetarian.

Just recently we saw two firsts for this strategy of reducing meat consumption: Baltimore became the first city to start serving 100 percent vegetarian meals one day a week in public schools, and across the pond the city of Ghent in Belgium has become the first to officially endorse meatless Thursdays. The momentum continues to build. As well, San Francisco's Board of Supervisors unanimously passed a resolution urging restaurants, stores, and schools to join in Meatless Mondays, and the state of Michigan declared a "Michigan Meatout Day."

Many signs suggest that as a society we may be about to reach a tipping point in our relationship with food. Today fully 10 percent of adults in the U.S.—well over 20 million individuals—say they largely follow a "vegetarian-inclined" diet. More importantly, 12 million others are "definitely interested" in going veg in the future.

More and more health-care institutions and concerned people are listening. The prestigious medical journal the *Lancet* has called upon the Western world to reduce its meat consumption by 10 percent, and thirty-two U.S. hospitals have committed to reduce their meat purchases by 20 percent through their participation in the Balanced Menu Challenge, an initiative of the nonprofit group Health Care Without Harm.

Today fully ten percent of adults in the U.S.—well over 20 million individuals—say they largely follow a "vegetarian-inclined" diet. More importantly, 12 million others are "definitely interested" in going veg in the future. Perhaps most promising are the changes evident among young people: multiple studies by the dining service giant Aramark have shown that approximately 25 to 30 percent of college students consider vegetarian meals at dining halls "very important" to them.

Demographic statistics are helpful in understanding the potential for change, but it's important not to forget that no matter how big a social phenomenon gets, change happens one person at a time. Take someone like Jack. A few years after finishing his law degree, Jack was at a dinner party with friends of friends. His hosts were in a "mixed marriage," an omnivore and a vegan, and the conversation went to food and problems in factory farming. Jack didn't have much to say (his hosts never knew the chain of events they initiated) but when he got home that evening he put three words into his Internet browser search field: *factory*, *farming*, and *video*.

It didn't take long for Jack to realize he didn't want to support what the meat industry had become. It was a gut response for Jack. The suffering he saw made him terribly uncomfortable, and he made a resolution: tomorrow I will eat no animal products. Soon it was a week animal-product-free, then a month. By the end of his vegan month Jack was not only feeling more energetic but was feeling like his life, his choices, had a new meaning.

Co-workers began complimenting him on his having lost weight. Jack's recurrent problem with back pain, which had been getting worse for years, stopped for good. The biggest fan of his new diet was his new girlfriend, Melissa. Vegan

diets tend to promote better circulation, which is likely why
Jack's back pain subsided, but as Dr. Ornish explained in
Promise 3, the benefits of greater circulation don't stop
there.

Fast-forward a few years: Melissa and Jack are married,
and their vegan cooking has earned them a reputation as excellent hosts. Jack and Melissa had always been well-liked
people in their community and decided to have a dinner party
of their own one night, all vegan. It was the first of many. One
friend confessed to Jack that the first time Jack invited him
over for dinner, he made a point of grabbing a burger before
arriving (*not* a veggie burger). That same friend is now a committed Meatless Mondays man and makes sure to eat a light
lunch if he'll be eating dinner at Jack and Melissa's. "If I
could have vegan food like this every day," guests would in-
variably report, "it would be easy to go vegan."

Jack never preached. He just dished up the best food he
could and shared his story and knowledge when others asked.

Five years after Jack went vegan, a handful of people in
his social circle had joined him in adopting a plant-based
diet. Most people he knew didn't make a complete switch, but
virtually everyone in his social circle had acquired a new per-
spective on food. Just by knowing a vegan couple for a few
years, the idea of a totally animal-free diet had come to seem
natural to them. One couple he knew had learned from him
that the seventh edition of Dr. Benjamin Spock's *Baby and
Child Care* urged parents to feed their children a completely
vegan diet. The couple hadn't been willing to change their
own diet, but it felt wrong to them to pass on what they knew
was a bad, addictive habit. By the time their son Jonathan was

three, the whole family was vegan (admittedly Mom and Dad were pretty sloppy about it when Jonathan wasn't involved).

Let's imagine the possibilities of what might happen from here. Fast-forward another twenty-five years. Baby Jonathan is now completing a degree in public health, graduating with honors with the class of 2035. In 2050 Jonathan is appointed to a presidential commission to develop new government recommendations on diet. Jonathan has no idea where the knowledge originated, but, as a vegan, he grew up knowing that he couldn't rely on U.S. government recommendations for diet because of the undue influence of factory farm corporations.

Sadly, the present structure of agribusiness still makes some of the most unhealthy food the most profitable to produce, exerting a corrupting influence on industry. Jonathan is hardly the most important person in shaping the presidential commission's recommendations (or the tenth most), but he does spearhead a successful effort to ensure that the next group of medical experts who will develop new government guidelines will be free of industry influence. It seems like a small thing, but looking back historians argue that the government guidelines produced in 2050 were the first to be viewed as scientifically credible by nutritional experts. The guidelines certainly made the health benefits of a plant-based diet clear to anyone who paid attention and, in the ensuing years, the percentage of people in the nation who went meatless hit a critical mass. The Western diet that had prevailed at the turn of the twenty-first century was soon regarded as a lesson in how food systems can go wrong.

Time travel being impossible, I'm sure you've surmised that Jack isn't a real person like the others whose stories

I've told in this book, but everything I've said about his story is true of more than one person I have known. And what couldn't be more real is the enormous influence we have on how other people eat—influences that can work in unexpected ways. Think about how your favorite foods became your favorite foods. Did you just find them on your own through vigorous taste-testing of whatever food you happen to see? Or were you introduced to the foods by other people?

What's also true about this story is that seeing a dramatic change in how a nation eats in one person's lifetime is eminently possible. This is a point that the food and farming advocacy group Farm Forward suggests we should keep in the forefront of our minds. "It is easy to forget," they point out,

> that over the last seventy years animal agriculture has changed more than in the last seven thousand. For example, 99.9 percent of the chickens we eat today are from breeds that were non-existent until the 1940s. And Americans today eat more than a hundred times as many chickens as we did in the 1930s. The sobering animal welfare, ecological, and public health problems these statistics point to are well known, but any historically-minded person will also see in them proof of how much and how fast dietary patterns can change. This generation will shape the future of food. The only question is whether we will raise our voice to shape a better future or let other voices—agribusiness, pharmaceutical companies, meat-industry lobbyists—rise out of our silence. The question is *what kind* of future we are shaping.

If dietary change seems hard, it's good to remember this history. As Farm Forward lays out, in modern times changing diets are the rule rather than the exception. And all of us can raise our voices about the shape of the future simply by changing how we raise our forks.

You can't know how your choices will ripple out into the world, but when it comes to food you can be sure the ripple effect is multiplying the impact of your choices. Even more, you can know that you are alive at a moment when change isn't just desirable, but necessary.

We are not only at a tipping point but also at a critical turning point. Beyond reaffirming that animal agriculture is the chief contributor of greenhouse gases, the latest United Nations report on climate change concludes that there is simply no other way to prevent the potentially catastrophic impacts of climate change other than for the world to move in the direction of plant-based diets. The report explains, "A substantial reduction of impacts would only be possible with a substantial worldwide diet change." This means that the choices we make today will be decisive ones in shaping the future. It means our choices matter.

Imagine

The possibility for change is immense. Consider the case of soy foods, which virtually always replace animal products in American diets. In 1992 the FDA made it legal for soy producers to indicate the link between consuming their product and reduction in heart disease risk. This modest move by the government and changing consumer demands led U.S. sales for soy foods to multiply by fourteen-fold in the next sixteen years—from $300 million to more than $4 billion. Soy milk, a relatively obscure beverage when I was born, is now present in more than one in ten American households, and some industry executives are expecting that number to triple in coming decades. The point is not that soy-based meat and dairy alternatives are the only or best ones but simply that there is enormous potential for positive change.

Imagine what's possible. As more and more people choose veganism, economies of scale will further lower costs and increase the variety and quality of meat and dairy alternatives. A cycle will follow in which food innovations and the increasing number of people going vegan will mutually reinforce each other. Soon that long row of animal flesh at the back of the grocery store will be occupied by varieties of tofu, tempeh, seitan, and other meat alternatives. Entire new industries will be created: new micro "dairies" will produce regional faux cheeses; demand for a more diverse variety of fruits and vegetables will drive new, more sustainable, and fairer trade agreements between nations; free from the stench and pathogens that surround meat production, a new generation of farmers will produce their crops in closer proximity to their neighbors.

Soy milk, a relatively obscure beverage when I was born, is now present in more than one in ten American households, and some industry executives are expecting that number to triple in coming decades.

People's quality of life and length of life will increase. Health insurance companies will start to give deep discounts to those who avoid meat and dairy and health-care costs will plummet, driving growth in businesses of all sizes. Animal agriculture will no longer have the political power to pollute waterways with near impunity. Deforestation will begin to reverse as less land is needed. Climate change will slow. Headlines once filled with news of emerging super-pathogens and oil spills will be replaced with reports on the decreasing number of foodborne illnesses and reduced reliance on fossil fuel. As people see the changes their generation helped create, a sense of empowerment will replace frustration. Healthier, safer, more ecologically balanced, and more inspired, future generations will take on new challenges with a confidence. We will learn to more fully realize our human potential.

If Only a Small Percentage . . .

Even if only a modest percentage of people move in the direction of a vegan diet, it will be a game changer. Consider the health-care costs directly attributable to meat. As we saw in Promise 5, the health-care costs of heart disease alone, which can be almost entirely eliminated through plant-based diets, are $500 billion annually. Even if the costs of this one disease were reduced by 30 percent it would amount to $150 billion dollars! What can you do with $150 billion that you are no longer spending on hospital bills? According to a report prepared by the Political Economy Research Institute at the University of Massachusetts, a $150 billion investment in green infrastructure would create 1.7 million green jobs. That's just one possibility, though.

Every American who switches from a typical U.S. diet to a vegan one has an extraordinary impact. They reduce their consumption of fossil fuels by more than 80 percent, cutting their carbon emissions by 3,000 pounds annually. According to a University of Chicago study, if Americans reduced their meat consumption by only 20 percent it would be as if everyone in the nation switched from a standard sedan to an ultra-efficient hybrid. By going vegetarian you will save three acres of land, save 2,700 pounds of soil from erosion, and save 95,000 gallons of water every year, year after year.

Even if we Americans reduced our meat consumption by only 5 percent (eating approximately one fewer meat dish a week), that would free up 7.5 million tons of grain, enough to feed the 25 million Americans who go hungry each day. And as we saw in Promise 7, if 10 percent of the world population gave up meat, it would be enough to feed the estimated billion people who go hungry annually. Tipping point or no, how we respond to our cravings for meat will have a global force.

Of course, for the animals who suffer on today's factory farms we don't need to calculate complex statistics to imagine how much our dietary choices matter. Even a single individual going vegan saves the lives of about 28 chickens and turkeys and 240 sea animals annually. If over time your influence ripples out to a thousand people and they too go veg, their diet will collectively save an additional 140 cows and 400 pigs *every year*. According to the Humane Society of the United States, if every American reduced his or her meat consumption by just 10 percent that would be enough to save roughly 1 billion animals from miserable lives annually. If that 10 percent reduction was maintained, in a bit more than a century more animal lives would be saved than the total number of human beings who have ever walked the earth.

Even if Americans ate just one fewer meat dish a week, that would free up 7.5 million tons of grain, enough to feed the 25 million Americans who go hungry each day. If 10 percent of the world population gave up meat, it would be enough to feed the estimated billion people who go hungry annually.

When we poll vegetarians and ask why they have chosen their diet, animal welfare concerns are the most commonly given response—about 54 percent of people give this reason (almost the same, 53 percent, cite health). For me animal suffering is one of the most compelling reasons to go vegan, but for others it is the least important. I recently had lunch with a well-known human rights activist. She had heard I was a human rights advocate, too, and I explained that I am, but I'm actually better known as an animal protection advocate. She looked dejected. The expression on her face said silently what she soon asked me. How can I care so much about animals when so many humans are suffering? How can I spend my time advocating vegetarianism when I could be speaking about the great issues of human rights? I understood. But I also wondered: *Why do so many smart and caring people seem to think that compassion is a competition?* As if caring about suffering anywhere, in any form, weren't a natural part of being a caring person! As if good deeds didn't lead to more good deeds! And if we can't get the little things right, how can we stand a chance at getting the really big things right?

Beyond the obvious—that a vegetarian diet is one of the best ways to help the global poor—it's worth remembering that calls for conscious eating are also calls for human morality and responsible stewardship. This is why Mahatma Gandhi, probably the single individual most responsible for the birth of a modern state, famously argued that the moral progress of nations can be judged by the way they treat their animals. Gandhi spent his life laboring on behalf of poor and oppressed people, but he also advocated plant-based diets and saw that true compassion does not ignore suffering, whether the suffering one is a different color or a different species. Gandhi knew that compassion is indeed a muscle that grows with use. Love of humanity and concern for animal suffering are a part of the same fabric of caring.

Compassion is a muscle that grows with use.

Being a veganist is as much about caring for yourself as it is caring for others, as much about concern for humanity as it is about concern for the earth and its creatures. In the end, a vegan diet lets us sow seeds of peace on many levels. This is what is so inspiring about the veganist challenge. The ultimate promise of a plant-based diet is that it will utterly transform our personal health even as it heals the world around us.

We are a generation that senses something big on the horizon. We have been longing for meaning, hungering for a sense of empowerment, for the ability to be the game changers we know this world needs. And here, right in front of us—on our plates, actually—is the means to make that splendid leap. And when we make that leap within ourselves, overcoming all the little obstacles and attachments, we take the world right along with us. We become the very hope we were looking for.

Afterword:

Making the Shift

MAKING A FUNDAMENTAL CHANGE TO YOUR DIET CAN BE OVER-whelming. And that's why I so often recommend *leaning in* to a new way of eating and not trying to make too many changes at once. As you might have read in my other books, I've been working on improving myself for quite some time. It's been a long process of pushing myself past my comfort zones and into healthier ways of living, and nothing has come overnight for me. There have been times when I "got" something readily, like an epiphany that felt right in my gut, but that doesn't necessarily mean the ensuing changes happened easily. There has always been a process of becoming conscious of where I need to change, and then getting there. Think of a bad relationship: You know it's not right for you anymore. You know it's damaging your self-esteem, or at the very least, is not in alignment with your soul's truth. You know there must be a better way of living, but you just don't know how to get out of what you've grown so accustomed to.

And the thing is, if you don't make a move, years can be lost and you lose precious opportunities to really thrive physically, emotionally, and spiritually. You may never know how great your life could have been, how much you could have really shone and made your mark.

It's the same with eating. We see a better way, but it's just a matter of getting there. As I outlined in *Quantum Wellness*, there are four simple steps that are quite powerful. By taking these steps, you set the process—any process of growth and self improvement—in motion.

1. **Listen and learn.** Keep eating what you are eating, all the while educating yourself on the effects of that food. Don't go to sleep; stay awake and alert. Read books about the nutritional benefits of a plant-based diet; watch videos online of animals being slaughtered. It will clarify things for you, and you will have loads of information to answer what people will inevitably question you about ("Don't you need to eat meat to get protein?" "Don't you think animals are meant to be food?"). Informing yourself will create enthusiasm and kick-start the process of change.

2. **Set an intention.** You may not know exactly how to get there, but you can lean in the direction of how you want to be. Say to yourself, "I want to be a person who lives consciously and eats healthfully. I want to look in the mirror and like what I see. I want to feel full of energy and apply that

energy to a meaningful life." After I'd read a few books on how animal protein was bad for me and watched some behind-the-scenes video of animals being raised in terrible conditions, I knew I wanted to be vegan. That was my intention. But because it was so radically different from how I currently ate, I couldn't get there in one leap. I just held on to that vision of myself; I had set an intention.

3. **Come up with a plan**. Well, as my grandmother always said, "Hell is paved with good intentions!" An intention is only the beginning. Next you need a plan on how to make things happen. In my case, I made a grocery list of new items I wanted to check out—new meat alternatives that looked and tasted like the favorite foods I'd been accustomed to. I went through websites and cookbooks and picked out a few recipes that looked easy and tasty. I searched for restaurants in my area that catered to vegetarians, or that had a vegan entrée on the menu. By coming up with a plan, you solidify your intention. It starts looking doable, and a momentum starts.

4. **Make the move**. This is when you just jump in. You simply take a step. No pressure, no hurry. Just a step. I began sampling different foods, inviting friends over for tastings. I kept a journal on how I felt and looked (I lost weight, my skin cleared up, and my eyes seemed more clear), and I was further energized by what I was seeing.

* * *

I'm not sure exactly how long the whole process was for me—but it was definitely not overnight. It was over the course of a couple of years, but that doesn't mean it has to take that long for you. I gave up one animal at a time, and found my footing slowly and surely. In that way, I leaned in to the life I wanted for myself, and things even took on a life of their own. (Now I'm an author on the subject; who knew?)

That's what I suggest to you. Take it one step at a time; stay curious and actively seek out new products and menu ideas, and you will find that there is a whole world of hearty, delicious food out there that does absolutely no harm—not to other living creatures, not to the planet, not to your health.

Some people dread the switch because they're so afraid of feeling deprived. And if switching over to a plant-based diet meant only *eliminating* animal foods, that's exactly what you'd feel. Not to mention hungry, dissatisfied, left out, and at a loss. People who try this route often feel like they're subsisting on side dishes, always longing for something more. Try that, and the white-knuckling willpower it would take would inevitably give way to temptation, and back you'd go to the burgers and fries. That's where "crowding out" comes in.

"Crowding out" is a term used in nutritional circles to describe how to eat in a healthy way without giving yourself the chance to feel hungry. You literally crowd out junk and bad food by adding in healthy foods throughout the day so that you're always satisfied. When you eat the veganist way, you eat nutrient-dense and fiber-rich foods, which satisfy your body's cravings and leave you feeling fulfilled and content.

Your body feels nutritionally satisfied, and there's no room left over for feeling deprived.

Those old bad habits literally get crowded out by better ones.

Tips for Making the Switch

1. Begin by leaving off one animal at a time. I suggest that you start by giving up eating all birds—chicken, turkey, and duck. As Alec Baldwin says in his *Meet Your Meat* video, "Chickens are probably the most abused animals on the face of the planet." The numbers factor is worth noting, too: In the U.S., we kill 100 times more chickens than pigs, and 200 times more chickens than cattle. If your concern is cruelty, drop poultry first.

So you can get used to not relying on poultry to round out your meals, work in some alternative vegetarian meats. I love Gardein (they have a great product that looks and tastes very much like chicken, while other products in their line are akin to pork and beef), which is found in most supermarket freezers and in the refrigerated section of Whole Foods and other health food stores. You can use their "chick'n" patties or scallopini to make the recipes you're used to making with animal chicken. For Thanksgiving, Gardein makes a great vegan turkey that can be found in the frozen foods section or ordered ahead of time through your local health food store. There are other vegan versions of turkey which you can find at health food stores, Trader Joe's, and even some of the bigger supermarkets, just look in the freezer section.

Tip: You may need a few weeks or a few months between each step; you will most likely know when it's time to push yourself to let go of another animal in your diet.

After you've found your footing and gotten used to one fewer animal in your meal plans, take out another. If you decide to give up red meat next, try chili with beans rather than chili con carne; instead of tacos with ground beef, try them with Smart Ground meatless crumbles. Gardein makes a great product called Beefless Tips, in the frozen section, that you can use to make dishes like beef stew and beef stroganoff, and they're great for stir-frys as well. Trader Joe's also makes fantastic meatballs that you can put into spaghetti or on a sandwich. They can be found in the freezer section of your local market. There are meat-free cold cuts, which make great sandwiches, and even kids don't seem to notice the difference. And you can do just about anything with tofu or seitan, too, so experiment with your traditional recipes by simply replacing the meat with a veg protein.

2. **Instead of pork bacon or sausage, discover all the wonderful veggie versions. They vary in taste and texture, so keep experimenting with brands until you find the ones you like the most. One of my favorite weekend meals is scrambled tofu with onions and sun-dried tomatoes, with veggie bacon on the side. It fulfills my traditional longing for a**

hearty "scramble" on a lazy weekend day without all the fuss.

3. Substitute tempeh, which is cultured soy, for tuna fish. Tempeh is high in protein and fiber, low in fat and can be mixed with vegan mayo and relish, with some nori (seaweed) crumbled in for a great tunalike salad to spread on crackers or fold into a sandwich.

4. Take weekend jaunts to the health food store and farmers' market so you can pick out new foods to get excited about. Try tamari-roasted almonds or dried apples or hummus; find ripe avocados and mangos and radishes to put in your salad. Pick up a spaghetti squash and see how delicious and easy it is to make (just bake it in the oven with some olive oil, and then shred it for a hearty side dish or add tomato sauce, to make another version of pasta!).

5. And while you're at it, try eating only natural sugars like stevia or brown rice syrup instead of the ones that will fatigue you and cause you to gain weight. Opt for sparkling water with a squeeze of lime or a bit of pomegranate juice rather than sugary sodas or juices (fruit juices spike your blood sugar and send you on an insulin roller coaster, even though the sugar is natural). Choose healthy treats made with whole grains and good quality sweeteners rather than the stuff that will get the old "addict" in you going. For instance, I switched to flax crackers with almond butter and agave

nectar drizzled on top from cookies or pastries. Making changes like these can inspire you to get healthy all around, and I encourage you to find where your weak spots are and fill them in with healthier alternatives. (My book *The Quantum Wellness Cleanse* is a good way to begin this process.)

6. Let go of eating eggs, too. There are far better (delicious, nutritious, and cruelty-free) alternatives readily available. For baking, use Ener-G egg replacer (a blend of tapioca starch, xanthan gum, and other natural ingredients) or, for each egg called for, just blend 1 tablespoon of ground flax seeds with 3 tablespoons water and microwave for 10 seconds. You will discover a whole world of vegan treats once you start looking for them!

7. For soups and sauces, there are wonderful vegetarian broths to replace chicken or beef broth.

8. Discover nondairy milks and cheeses. Dairy was the last thing I gave up, and it was the thing that I loved the most (until I learned all about the dairy cattle industry!). The hardest habit for me to break was my snack of cheese and crackers; I just loved the ritual of sitting down to something that was so familiar. But instead of letting myself feel deprived, I simply chose new snacks, like guacamole and chips, hummus with pita or cucumbers, nuts, nut spreads on flax crackers or rice cakes, or fruit.

Nondairy milks include soy, almond, rice, and hemp; you can get them in different flavors, sweetened or not. For lightening my tea and coffee, my absolute favorite is Silk Soy Creamer, because it's rich and thick and won't separate in hot beverages. Westsoy Crème de la Soy is also terrific. And there are wonderful nondairy ice creams that are as tasty as anything you grew up with. Great vegan cheeses can be used to make pizza and grilled cheese sandwiches, or sprinkle them over soups and mix into salads; just look for them next to the regular cheese in health food stores and some supermarkets. I like Daiya, which is made from tapioca. Some people think soy cheeses taste "odd," but I think they're terrific, and I've made many converts over the years. Nutritional yeast flakes, found at health food stores, are also great sprinkled over pasta instead of Parmesan, and they're loaded with B_{12} and protein.

9. When traveling, bring some dried fruits and nuts for the plane or between meetings. It's also not a bad idea to pack up leftovers from the night before in a "to go" box (save the ones you get from restaurant takeout) and bring them with you, or make a couple of sandwiches and a thermos of soup to have on hand. Wherever you are, you can always run into a supermarket to grab some fresh fruit, nut butter, or cut up veggies. Nearly every hotel serves oatmeal for breakfast—just ask room

service to have the kitchen make it with either water or soy milk rather than regular milk, which is their fallback preparation; you can sprinkle on your nuts and fruits if they don't have any to accompany the dish. Or you can ask for toast or a bagel with peanut butter and a fruit plate. The nicer hotels offer soy milk, but if you suspect there won't be any at the one you are going to, and your coffee won't be the same without cream, you can buy powdered nondairy creamer (not the old-fashioned hydrogenated kind; go to the health food store for it instead, and steer clear of anything with sodium caseinate in it, because that is a milk product). It's not really that tasty, but it'll do in a pinch. That said, be sure that the hotelier or airline hears your request for nondairy options, because when they hear enough noise, they will eventually respond.

I travel with small packets of protein powder in case I don't get enough whole foods to cover my nutritional needs while on the road; I shake it up in a bottle of water and pour in some ground flax seeds for fiber. Sometimes I even go back to the kitchen of the hotel and ask them to put my protein powder in with some water and bananas and blueberries and blend it all up. I tell them they can charge me for it, as it's worth it to me to eat something healthy rather than gorge on bread if that's all they have that's vegan. Another fun snack for the road is vegetarian jerky, which is high in protein.

10. When choosing which restaurants to go to, check out the local ethnic eateries, because they will usually have more interesting and delicious vegetarian and vegan options. Indian, Mexican, Thai, Ethiopian, Lebanese, Chinese, and Japanese cuisines all have a strong plant-based orientation. At fancier restaurants, I often mention that I'm a vegan when making my reservation. Restaurant kitchens get very busy, so if you order something vegan upon arrival the cooks may be too frenzied to whip up anything interesting; but if you give them advance notice, the chef is usually more than happy to have something in store for you when you arrive. If you go to more all-American sorts of restaurants, you can always ask them to put everything vegetable/bean/legume/potato on a plate for a vegetarian smorgasbord. Most places also have pasta primavera (pasta with veggies), but you don't want to eat pasta every time you go out. Try to resist filling up on empty carbs like bread. If you take that route rather than eating healthy, nutritious foods, you will only bloat up, gain weight, and lose energy. If they simply don't offer fresh vegetables, grains, or fruits, do the best you can until you get home and can take control of your menu. Oh, and ask for olive oil rather than butter; it's delicious on bread or potatoes with a little pinch of salt.

11. If you are invited to a dinner party, let your host know ahead of time that you are vegan and

ask if she would like you to bring a dish or two. It will most likely make for interesting dinner conversation, so bring enough to share! If it's a barbecue, bring over some veggie dogs and burgers and vegan cheese, so that you can join in with everyone else. Don't worry about offending anyone; as long as you are gracious and don't preach about what anyone else should eat, everything will be fine. And if it's not, and your host seems prickly, chalk it up to it being nothing you can change. You can't make everyone happy, but you can be kind and informative (if asked) and people will eventually come to understand your new way of eating (if not join you!).

12. Try to eat a few servings of veggies every day, whether as side dishes, in salads, or as centers to the meal (like stuffed butternut squash). When you eat a wide variety of colorful, fresh veggies, you guarantee yourself lots of fiber and much of your needed nutrition. Enjoy lentils, chickpeas, beans, tofu, seitan, and tempeh, and meat alternatives like Gardein for your main sources of protein, but remember, protein is in just about everything, so if you are eating a varied plant-based diet, you will most likely be getting plenty. And enjoy your fruit—pears, strawberries, figs—as snacks or condiments; you won't need sugar to satisfy your sweet tooth when you enjoy fruits regularly.

13. One of my favorite ways of getting in a couple doses of fruits and veggies is to throw them into a smoothie. I start with a base of coconut water or nondairy milk and protein powder—I like Solaray Soytein, Life's Basics, or Vegn because they are not sweetened with anything that will spike blood sugar—then add in blueberries or raspberries. The kicker is the cup of frozen broccoli; you can't even taste it when it goes in frozen, so even kids will go for it.

14. Steer clear of junk foods like chips and cookies and sweets (well, at least don't make a habit of eating them!) so that you keep your energy high and your cravings low (remember: junk begets cravings for more junk). Just getting animal products out of your diet alone won't make you thrive; you still need to crowd in nutritious foods while saying no to empty calories.

15. Don't make yourself (or the waiter!) crazy about foods that may have less than 2 percent of something animal in them. For instance, don't interrogate your server to make sure there is no milk in the bread or insist that your veggie burger is not on the same grill as a steak. You don't want to give the impression that vegans are hard to please!

When you are adding in all these delicious and nutritious foods, you won't miss the things you are taking out. In fact, you will be glad they are out of your diet, and out of your body. If you backslide and eat something you wished you hadn't, don't worry about it. Note how you feel, and plan for what you will do the next time you are tempted. The trick is to re-place—crowd out—what you no longer want to eat so that you never feel deprived, and fill your home with delicious food so that there is always something healthy on hand.

As you become a veganist (or vegan-ish), your tastes will also evolve. In fact, your taste buds themselves will change; they will adjust to the cleaner, purer flavors. Your skin will look brighter, you will shed weight if you need to, and you will im-prove your overall health. Your energy, too, will begin to lift be-cause you will be getting good nutrition while at the same time avoiding all the problems that go along with rich, fatty, prob-lematic animal protein. The more you lean in to healthy eating, the more you will be supported by feelings of well-being—not just in your body, but in your mind and soul as well.

Frequently Asked Questions, Answered by the Doctor

THERE ARE SO MANY MYTHS AND MISINFORMATION AROUND FOOD, so I suspect you might have a question or two. Here are the ones most commonly asked, answered by Dr. Neal Barnard of the Physicians Committee for Responsible Medicine. And if you have more questions, you might want to consult their website at www.pcrm.org.

1. Where do I get iron if not from red meat?

The most healthful sources of iron are "greens and beans." That is, green leafy vegetables and anything from the bean group. These foods also bring you calcium and other important minerals.

Vegetables, beans, and other foods provide all the iron you need. In fact, studies show that vegetarians and vegans tend to get more iron than meat eaters. Vitamin C increases iron absorption. Meanwhile, dairy products reduce iron absorption significantly.

To go into a little more detail, there are actually two forms of iron. Plants have nonheme iron, which is more absorbable when the body is low in iron and less absorbable when the body already has enough iron. This allows the body to regulate its iron balance. On the other hand, meats have heme iron, which barges right into your bloodstream whether you need it or not. The problem is that many people have too much iron stored in their bodies. Excess iron can spark the production of free radicals that accelerate aging, increase the risk of heart disease, and cause other problems.

So while it's important to avoid anemia, you also do not want to be iron overloaded. It's probably best to have your hemoglobin on the low end of the normal range. If your energy is good and your hemoglobin and hematocrit are at the low end of normal, that is likely the best place to be.

Having said that, you will want your doctor to review your laboratory results and to track them over time. If your hemoglobin and hematocrit are dropping, that may be a sign of blood loss. That can be from benign causes, such as menstrual flow, but can also reflect more dangerous health issues, such as intestinal bleeding.

2. What is the best source of calcium, and how does it compare with dairy?

The same green leafy vegetables and legumes that provide iron are also good sources of calcium, for the most part, and absorption is typically better from these sources than from dairy products. One common exception is spinach, which has a great deal of calcium, but it's absorption is poor. But broccoli, brussels sprouts, kale, and other common greens have highly absorbable calcium.

If you like, you can also use calcium-fortified products such as breakfast cereals and juices, although these products provide more concentrated calcium than is necessary. It pays to put some thought into keeping your bones healthy. Studies have shown that the following factors are helpful in building and maintaining strong bones:

- **Getting plenty of exercise.** Studies have concluded that physical exercise is the key to building strong bones (it's more important than any other factor). For example, a study published in the *British Medical Journal* that followed 1,400 men and women over a fifteen-year period found that exercise may be the best protection against hip fractures and that "reduced intake of dietary calcium does not seem to be a risk factor." And at Penn State University, researchers found that bone density is significantly affected by how much exercise girls get during their teen years, when 40 to 50 percent of their skeletal mass is formed.

- **Getting enough vitamin D.** If you don't spend any time in the sun (about fifteen minutes on the face and arms each day is enough), be sure to take a supplement or eat fortified foods.

- **Eliminating animal protein.** For a variety of reasons, animal protein causes calcium losses.

- **Limiting salt intake.** Sodium tends to cause the body to lose calcium in the urine.

- **Eating plenty of fruits and vegetables.** People who eat lots of vegetables and fruits are less likely to have bone breaks. Part of the reason may be that they contain vitamin C, which is essential for building collagen, the underlying bone matrix.

- **Not smoking.** Studies have shown that women who smoke one pack of cigarettes a day have 5 to 10 percent less bone density at menopause than nonsmokers.

3. Is it healthy for a pregnant or nursing mother to eat a plant-based diet? How about kids?

According to the American Dietetic Association:

> Well-planned vegan and other types of vegetarian diets are appropriate for all stages of the life-cycle including during pregnancy, lactation, infancy, childhood, and adolescence. Vegetarian diets offer a number of nutritional benefits including lower levels of saturated fat, cholesterol, and animal protein as well as higher levels of carbohydrates, fiber, magnesium, potassium, folate, antioxidants such as vitamins C and E, and phytochemicals. Vegetarians have been reported to have lower body mass indices than nonvegetarians, as well as lower rates of death from ischemic heart disease, lower blood cholesterol levels, lower blood pressure, and lower rates of hypertension, type 2 diabetes, and prostate and colon cancer.
>
> —American Dietetic Association position paper on vegetarian and vegan diets

In the seventh edition of Dr. Benjamin Spock's *Baby and Child Care*—the last edition published during Dr. Spock's lifetime—he spelled out some good advice for children's diets. He recommended that children be served plant-based diets—vegan diets—and that, to deal with finicky eaters, the best approach was not to arm-wrestle with children, but rather to simply find healthful foods they will eat. For example, children may not like cooked spinach, but they will like fresh spinach as part of a salad. They often are not keen on more exotic vegetables, but they are fine with corn, carrots, green beans, etc.

Virtually all children like the following:

Legumes: baked beans (okay to add cut-up veggie hot dogs), lentil soup, split pea soup, peas, bean burritos, bean tacos

Vegetables: carrots, green beans, vegetable soup, salads

Grains: rice, whole grain bread, oatmeal, cold cereals with soy milk or rice milk, corn, vegan pizza, spaghetti with chunky tomato sauce

Fruits: apples, bananas, and all others

Meat analogues: veggie burgers, veggie hot dogs, etc. The soy-based ones have a cancer-preventing effect for girls, and are healthful for all children.

It is also important to provide a pediatric multiple vitamin.

PCRM has a book called *Healthy Eating for Life: For Children*, which is very detailed on veganism and kids.

4. Do I need to take any particular vitamins or minerals because of eating this way?

Actually, vegans generally have better overall vitamin intake, compared with meat eaters. Meat has essentially no vitamin C and is low in many other vitamins as well. In contrast, vegetables, fruits, and legumes (beans, peas, and lentils) are vitamin-rich. In controlled studies, people switching to vegan diets typically increase their intake of several vitamins, and reduce their intake of the undesirables—saturated fat and cholesterol, in particular.

Even so, two vitamins deserve special comment:

Vitamin B_{12} is made, not by plants or animals, but by bacteria. Animal products contain B_{12} made by the bacteria in their intestinal tracts. A more healthful source is any common multiple vitamin. B_{12} supplements are also widely available.

Vitamin D normally comes from exposure to the sun. About fifteen minutes of direct sunlight on your face and arms each day gives you all the vitamin D you need. However, if you are indoors much of the day or live in an area where sunlight is limited, it is important to take a supplement. Any common multivitamin is fine. Most foods have little or no vitamin D. Certain fish contain some vitamin D, but they also harbor cholesterol, mercury, and other things you don't want. Surprisingly, mushrooms (for example, shiitakes and chanterelles) contain vitamin D. Five dried shiitakes provide roughly 5 micrograms of vitamin D. You'll also find it in fortified soy milk.

Nowadays, some health authorities recommend high vitamin D intakes—up to 2,000 IU (50 micrograms) per day, because of its reputed cancer-fighting properties. To get there, you'll need to take a vitamin D supplement. Vitamin D_2 (ergocalciferol) is plant-derived, while vitamin D_3, or chole-calciferol, typically comes from lanolin in sheep's wool.

5. How much protein do I need and where is the best place to get it?

A plant-based diet easily provides all the protein the body needs. There is no need for meat, dairy products, or eggs for protein, and you are better off without them. Vegetables, grains, and beans give you plenty of protein, even if you are active and athletic. And there is no need to eat these foods in any special combinations. The normal mixtures of food people choose from day to day easily satisfy protein needs.

For people who like technical details, protein is made up of amino acids. Each amino acid molecule is like a bead, and many amino acids together make up the protein chain. There are many different amino acids, and all of the essential ones are found in plants.

And by all means, do not fret about protein grams or feel any need to count them. But if you are interested in the numbers, simply divide your body weight (in pounds) by three. That gives you an approximation of the number of grams of protein your body needs, plus a margin for safety. So, for example, for a person who weighs 120 pounds, 40 grams of protein is more than enough on a daily basis. Some experts believe that the actual amount of protein required is actually much less than this figure.

The bottom line is to have a healthful mix of vegetables, beans, whole grains, and fruits, and protein takes care of itself.

6. What's the scoop on soy?

This bears repeating, so that you can feel really clear. Soy products have been around for thousands of years and are a dietary staple in many regions of Asia. Research has shown that people in these regions have lower rates of heart disease, breast and prostate cancer, fewer hip fractures and fewer hot flashes. In addition, dozens of clinical studies have indicated the health benefits of diets rich in soy.

Some have raised the question as to whether soy has untoward effects. Happily, these concerns have been set aside. Girls who consume soy products in adolescence have about a 30 percent reduction in breast cancer risk as adults. Women previously diagnosed with breast cancer have a significantly greater survival if they include soy in their diets, compared with women who tend not to use soy products.

However, if a person is uncertain or simply does not want to include soy, I always remind them that a vegan diet does not mean joining the Soy Promotion Society. A vegan diet can mean many things: a Latin American tradition with beans, rice, and tortillas; a Mediterranean tradition emphasizing vegetables, pasta, beans, and fruit. Soy products come from an Asian tradition and are totally optional.

7. What if I think I'm allergic to soy?

Again, eating a diverse diet of whole grains, beans and legumes, fruits and vegetables will give you everything you require in terms of protein. As for allergies, in some cases, they will change over time. For example, it is very common for children to have allergies that disappear as they get older, and that occurs in adulthood, too. Also, quite often, allergic

responses diminish when people stop consuming dairy products. For example, a person who is allergic to cats or has
asthma symptoms in response to pollen will find that these
symptoms diminish when they leave dairy products aside.

8. Where can I get my omega-3s if not from fish or fish oil?

ALA (alpha-linolenic acid) is a basic omega-3 fat that can be
converted in the body to the other omega-3s the body needs.
ALA occurs in small amounts in beans, vegetables, and
fruits, and this should be all the body needs. If more is de-
sired, it is also found in walnuts, soy products, and, in high
concentration, in flax seeds and flax oil. If these are used,
there is no need for more than minimal amounts.

If you are looking for more, for whatever reason, health
food stores sell vegan omega-3 supplements.

9. Sometimes eating lots of vegetables, beans, or soy products gives me uncomfortable gas; how do you avoid this?

The problem with gassiness can often be found with beans.
They should not be excluded from the diet, however, because
they are great sources of protein, calcium, and iron, among
other nutrients. But if you are new to beans, it is good to have
them in small portions and always very well cooked. A well-
cooked bean is very soft, with no hint of crunchiness. As time
goes on, your digestive tract adjusts, so a bean that may cause
a problem today may be better tolerated later on.

Also, cruciferous vegetables can cause indigestion for
some people. The answer is simply to cook them well. This

group includes broccoli, cauliflower, brussels sprouts, kale, and cabbage, among others. It is common for people to eat them raw or only slightly cooked, but they can easily cause gassiness or bloating. Cook them well, and the problem usually disappears. Later on, you can experiment again with less-cooked vegetables.

On the good side, rice is very easily digested, and a great food to emphasize. Brown rice is best. Also, cooked green, yellow, and orange vegetables are very easily digested.

Fruit vary. Some people do very well with raw fruit; others have more difficulty at first. If you are new to any particular fruit, you might have smaller servings at first, then gradually increase.

Three Weeks of Meals

Since so many people ask me, "What do you eat if not meat, dairy, and eggs?" I've prepared a list of what a few weeks of eating looks like in my home or when I'm at a restaurant. You can use the cookbooks and recipe websites listed in Resources to flesh out your shopping list and find things that appeal to you; or do like I do and guess at how something can be made and get creative! You can get fancier or go simpler according to your lifestyle needs.

Monday (Week One)
  Breakfast: steel-cut oatmeal, sliced bananas, walnuts, rice milk
  Lunch: whole grain pasta with veggie sausages, sun-dried tomatoes, broccoli; salad
  Dinner: seitan Parmesan with tomato sauce, green beans, mashed potatoes
Tuesday
  Breakfast: bagel with Earth Balance butter

LUNCH: sandwich with vegan cold cuts, nondairy cheese, avocado, pickles; tomato soup

DINNER: tacos with "meat" crumbles, nondairy cheese, guacamole; salad

WEDNESDAY

BREAKFAST: bagel with almond or peanut butter

LUNCH: split pea soup with tempeh bacon, (nondairy) cheesy toast; salad

DINNER: stuffed butternut or acorn squash with tofu; sautéed collard greens

THURSDAY

Breakfast: frozen waffles with Earth Balance butter, maple syrup

LUNCH: black bean and soy cheese quesadilla with guacamole; salad

DINNER: pan-seared Gardein fillet with shiitake-mushroom sauce; mashed potatoes and braised brussels sprouts

FRIDAY

BREAKFAST: brown rice (I make several days' worth at a time), chopped dates, almonds, nondairy milk poured over

LUNCH: cabbage, thyme, and meatless ground beef soup; 7-grain garlic bread

DINNER: coconut curry tofu with whole grain wild rice and green beans

SATURDAY

BREAKFAST: brown rice with blueberries and almonds; hemp milk

LUNCH: smoked paprika pinto beans with quinoa and sautéed kale

Dinner: charred seitan skewers, wheat berries; chili broccoli

Sunday

Breakfast: whole grain pancakes and blueberries; tempeh bacon

Lunch: chili with pinto beans, tomatoes, peppers, and onions, soy sour cream; salad

Dinner: seitan Parmesan (seitan fillets with melted nondairy cheese, tomato sauce), collard greens, mashed potatoes

Monday (Week Two)

Breakfast: soy yogurt with blueberries and almonds

Lunch: oven-roasted stuffed zucchini flowers on top of fig and walnut salad

Dinner: pasta with porcini mushrooms; salad

Tuesday

Breakfast: quinoa (I make a big batch that will last a few days), chopped dates, almonds, nondairy milk poured over

Lunch: flax-seed and whole grain pizza crust with classic margherita topping

Dinner: portobello mushroom and cannelloni bean burger with roasted peppers and sautéed Swiss chard

Wednesday

Breakfast: smoothie with avocado, agave, lime, and mint

Lunch: beefless stew (Gardein beefless tips); salad

Dinner: veggie hot dogs with sauerkraut; salad

Thursday

Breakfast: breakfast cookies (recipe in *Quantum Wellness Cleanse*)

LUNCH: tempeh tuna salad over greens; crackers

DINNER: Mediterranean platter of hummus, baba ganoush, tabouleh, pita bread

FRIDAY

BREAKFAST: breakfast cookies

LUNCH: bean burrito with salsa and guacamole; salad

DINNER: grilled tempeh with fresh oranges, shallots, and garlic; mashed sweet potatoes, sautéed spinach

SATURDAY

BREAKFAST: scrambled tofu with onions and sun-dried tomatoes; tempeh bacon

LUNCH: vegetable gumbo with soy sausage; salad

DINNER: soba noodles with vegetables and tofu

SUNDAY

BREAKFAST: vegan French toast with strawberries

LUNCH: tostada with rice, beans, and avocado.

DINNER: pasta puttanesca with summer squash

When you are on the run, here are some quick suggestions:

MONDAY (WEEK THREE)

BREAKFAST: Clif Bar; apple

LUNCH: eggless tofu salad (buy prepared at health food store) on brown rice bread; prepared green salad

DINNER: frozen brown rice, microwaved†; organic black beans; brussels sprouts, microwaved

---

†Always be cautious when using a microwave. There are health implications to microwaving in plastic, so please do your research on this, and only use the microwave when there is no other choice.

Tuesday

> Breakfast: frozen oatmeal, microwaved; blueberries on top
>
> Lunch: MorningStar Farms Grillers Vegan Veggie Burger, wrapped in lettuce; sweet potato tortilla chips
>
> Dinner: Amy's Brown Rice, Black-Eyed Peas & Veggies Bowl

Wednesday

> Breakfast: soy yogurt; banana
>
> Lunch: veggie hot dogs on whole-wheat buns; prepared salad
>
> Dinner: soy cheeze pizza, from freezer section; salad

Thursday

> Breakfast: MorningStar Farms Sausage Patties on bagel with vegan cheese; fruit
>
> Lunch: Amy's Non Dairy Bean & Rice Burrito
>
> Dinner: frozen veggie stir-fry, microwaved; frozen brown rice, microwaved

Friday

> Breakfast: Amy's Mexican Tofu Scramble
>
> Lunch: organic vegetable soup; multigrain bread with Earth Balance butter
>
> Dinner: MorningStar Farms Hickory BBQ Riblets; frozen vegetables

Saturday

> Breakfast: multibran cereal, almond milk, blueberries
>
> Lunch: frozen vegetable samosas; salad bar
>
> Dinner: Amy's Veggie Loaf with Mashed Potatoes & Veggies

SUNDAY

> BREAKFAST: organic frozen waffles with peanut butter; banana
>
> LUNCH: meatless deli slices on brown rice bread; organic blue corn tortilla chips
>
> DINNER: Kashi Frozen Tuscan Veggie Bake entrée; salad bar

Spend some time in the grocery store, going up and down the aisles, looking for new, fun, and creative foods that you may have overlooked when you only focused on animal products in your meal plans. There are many delicious, exciting, and nutritious foods available that are completely vegan and fulfilling, and many of them can be found at the deli prepared section of health food stores or in the freezer section of any grocery store. Again, whole foods like fresh vegetables and fruits, beans, and whole grains are best, but also try alternative plant-based meats to fulfill the traditional cravings for what you grew up loving.

Shopping List

HERE ARE SOME GREAT FINDS AND SHOPPING LIST IDEAS (SEARCH the aisles for more, these are just my favorites!) for three types of grocery stores, depending on convenience or what is available in your hometown.

"Big Chain" Grocery Store
FROZEN FOODS

Organics Organic Brown Rice (3 pouches, ready in 3 minutes)

Garden veggie mixes or veggie stir-frys

Organics organic frozen blueberries, organic frozen raspberries, organic frozen mangos

Gardein protein items—Chik'n Scallopini, pulled pork, BBQ skewers (my favorites!), breakfast patties

Boca items—Chik'n Patties and meatless products

Amy's Soy Cheeze Pizza and No Cheese Pizza

Amy's Baked Ziti Bowl; Brown Rice, Black-Eyed Peas & Veggies Bowl

Amy's gluten and dairy-free mac and cheese
Amy's Non Dairy Bean & Rice Burrito
Kashi Frozen Entrees Black Bean Mango, Tuscan Veggie
Bake

SOUPS

Organics Southwestern Black Bean Soup, or Butternut
Squash
Eating Right Vegetable Soup
Amy's Organic Chili, Black Bean, Low Fat
Annie Chun's Miso Soup Bowl

BREAKFAST/CEREAL

Bear Naked All Natural Granola
Cascadian Farm Organic Granola, Oats & Honey
Nature's Path Flax Plus Flakes
Nature's Path Flax Plus Organic Frozen Waffles
Organic steel-cut oats
Silk soy yogurt

FOR KIDS

Tofurky or Yves meatless deli slices
Annie's Honey Bunny Grahams
Organic B.R.A.T.—Banana, Rice & Applesauce
Tummy-Soothers
Newman's Own Fig Newmans (wheat-free and dairy-free)
Brown rice or whole-wheat spaghetti
Veggie hot dogs
Gardein Seven Grain Crispy Tenders (better than
chicken nuggets!)

MorningStar Farms Grillers Vegan Veggie Burgers
MorningStar Farms Grillers Chik'n Veggie Patties
Late July Organic Mini Bite Size Peanut Butter
     Sandwich Crackers

Snacks

Tortilla chips
Eating Right Barbeque Soy Crisps, Sea Salt Soy Crisps
Food Should Taste Good Sweet Potato Tortilla Chips
Clif Bars
Nuts: almonds, pecans, walnuts, pistachios
Fruit
Dried fruit (make sure there is no added sugar or corn
     syrup)
Popcorn

Ice Creams

Tofutti Cuties Vanilla and Mint Chocolate Chip Ice
     Cream Sandwiches
Tofutti Marry Me Dessert Bars
Ciao Bella sorbets

Trader Joe's
Frozen

TJ's Chickenless Nuggets
TJ's Organic Brown Rice (3 pouches, ready in 3 minutes)
TJ's Black Bean and Corn Enchiladas
TJ's Steelcut Oatmeal
MorningStar Farms Hickory BBQ Riblets

MorningStar Farms Grillers Vegan Veggie Burgers
Dr Praeger's California Veggie Burgers
Pad thai with tofu
Misto Alla Griglia Marinated Grilled Eggplant & Zucchini
Penne arrabbiata

REFRIGERATED SECTION

High Protein Organic Tofu and Organic Baked Tofu
Lightlife Organic Three Grain Tempeh
Tofurky Italian Sausages
Chicken-less Stuffed Cutlet
Eggless Egg Salad
Earth Balance Whipped Buttery Spread
Sweet potato spears
Asparagus (can be microwaved in package tray)
Brussels sprouts (can be microwaved in package bag)
Lentils—served hot or cold
Precut and washed carrots
Hummus
Prepared salads

SOUPS

Garden Patch Veggie Soup
Latin Black Bean Soup
Tasty Thai Green Curry
Indian Fare Punjab Eggplant, Dal Makhani
Mushroom Rice Noodle Soup Bowl

BREAKFAST

Milks: almond, hemp, rice, soy, oat
Natural toasted oat bran

Organic oats and flax
Organic Cinnamon Spice Oatmeal
Instant and regular organic steel-cut oats
Kashi 7 Whole Grain Puffs Cereal
Trader Joe's Fiber O's Cereal

KIDS

Tofutti Better Than Cream Cheese and bagel
Fruit with nut butter
Soy yogurt
Granola bars
Lightlife Smart Dogs (refrigerated)
Crinkled wedge potatoes (frozen)
TJ's Meatless Corn Dogs (frozen)
TJ's Meatless Meatballs (frozen)
TJ's Bean & Rice Burritos
TJ's Breadless Chickenless Nuggets
Toaster waffles (frozen)

GRAINS/BREADS

Organic brown-rice pasta (fusilli, penne)
Organic quinoa
Organic polenta
Whole-wheat couscous
Brown-rice bread

SNACKS

Root vegetable corn chips
Blue corn organic tortilla chips
Popcorn

Corn chip dippers
Nut butters (almond, peanut, sunflower seed)
Trail mixes
Nuts
Dried fruit
Organic brown-rice cakes
Dips and salsas
Kettle Corn
Salt & Pepper Crisps
Flax crackers
Wasa Crackers with nut butter and agave

DESSERTS/ICE CREAM

Tofutti Cuties
TJ's Sorbets
72% dark or bittersweet chocolate (any chocolate
    marked over 70% is nondairy, and you can now even
    find "milk" chocolate made from rice milk)
Vegan cookies
Soy Dream Soy Creams

Whole Foods/Health Food Stores
FROZEN

Bahama Rice Burger—Mediterranean and Original
Amy's Bistro Burger—gluten-free
Sunshine Veggie Burgers
Gardein frozen products (all vegan)
MorningStar Farms Hickory BBQ Riblets
MorningStar Farms Chick'n Strips
Nate's Meatless Meatballs

Nate's Meatless Nuggets
Amy's Bowls: Brown Rice, Black Eyed Peas & Veggies
Amy's Veggie Loaf with Mashed Potatoes and Veggies
Amy's Indian Vegetable Korma or Mattar Tofu
Amy's Enchilada or Burrito Especial

REFRIGERATED SECTION

Food for Life Sprouted Corn Tortillas
Mt Olive Falafel
Lightlife Smart Dogs
Tofurky Italian-style Deli Slices
Westsoy Baked Tofu, Italian-style
Gardein products

BREAKFAST/CEREAL

Nature's Path Frozen Waffles (Gluten-Free, Original,
    and Flax Plus)
Amy's Mexican Tofu Scramble

KIDS

Health Is Wealth Chicken-Free Vegan Nuggets and
    Patties
Ian's Mac & No Cheese (wheat-free and gluten-free)
Amy's Rice Macaroni & Soy Cheeze
Thai Kitchen Noodle kits

SNACKS

Garden Fresh Salsa
Clif Bars
Rice cakes

Dried fruit
Prepared hummus
Baba ganoush
Cascadian Farm Granola Bars
Sweet Potato Breakfast Pudding
Vegan chocolate mousse

NONDAIRY ICE CREAM

Purely Decadent
It's Soy Delicious
Rice Dream
Bliss (made from coconut milk)
Tempt (made from hemp milk)
Good Karma, Organic Rice Divine
Tofutti
Tofutti Cuties (ice cream sandwiches)

Stock Those Staples

Here are the basic foods I nearly always have on hand . . .

Proteins

Tofu: Tofu is soybean curd. It has very little flavor of its own, so it can be used in either savory or sweet dishes, and will take on the flavor of whatever sauce or seasoning you use. It's low in calories, cholesterol, and fat, and it's high in protein and iron. Find it near the cheese or the fresh-foods sections of markets.

Tempeh: Tempeh is made from cultured soybeans and formed into a sort of cake. It is easily digestible, has a nutty flavor, and is very high in protein, dietary fiber, and vitamins. It has a stronger flavor than tofu. It's usually found near the cheese section. It's a little pungent, and not everyone has a taste for it. But it's really healthy!

Seitan: Seitan is made from gluten, the protein part of wheat, and is chewy in texture. It is high in protein, very low in fat, and is extremely versatile in cooking. Nearly anything made with meat can be made with seitan instead. It's near the cheese or vegan section of your market.

Beans and legumes: They are high in protein, fiber, iron, and folic acid; they also have complex carbohydrates (the good kind!). You can keep them in your pantry for a while, and use them for bean salads, soups, and casseroles: black beans, lentils, chickpeas, lima beans, adzuki beans, black-eyed peas, edamame, fava beans, and many more. Canned are also fine!

Nuts and seeds/butter: They have plenty of fiber and antioxidants along with healthy monounsaturated fats; nuts and seeds go far in filling you up and making you feel satiated. Try almonds, cashews, walnuts, pecans, pistachios; almond butter, peanut butter, tahini, etc. Choose raw and unsweetened, with no salt. (I do love salted and roasted . . . but raw is better!)

Gardein Garden+Protein: These high-protein, center-of-the-plate meat alternatives are delicious and easy to prepare, as an entrée or an ingredient in a soup, stew, sandwich, or whatever. Gardein is my absolute favorite alternative meat, as it tastes so good and my meat-eating friends always love it. I recommend the Beefless Tips, which are great for stew or on a skewer with veggies, and the Chick'n Scallopini, which you can use in any way you would use chicken; it's highly versatile and easy to cook with. See www.gardein.com.

Tofurky: I love the Italian Deli Slices for sandwiches. They also make several flavors and styles of tempeh. And their holiday "turkey" looks like sliced turkey, so you can enjoy the feast along with everyone else at the table. See www.tofurky.com

Field Roast: These folks make two of my favorite products— Celebration Roast, which is a vegan "roast" with mushroom stuffing; it's a nice presentation for holiday or special events and great with a homemade sauce or gravy. Also their Field Roast Sausages are the best and come in several different flavors. I like the Italian and serve it with portabella mushrooms, red peppers, fennel root, tomatoes, and garlic over pasta. See www.fieldroast.com.

Nate's: Meatless Meatballs! Add them to a pasta sauce, or sauté; stick toothpicks in them and voilà, a delicious appetizer. Now you can add "Meatballs" to anything!

Starches

Whole grains: brown or wild rice, millet, quinoa, amaranth, buckwheat, corn

Sweet potatoes, yams, roasting potatoes

Flax crackers, rice cakes

Steel-cut oats and whole grain hot cereal mixes

Whole grain breads (try the sprouted ones, and go for gluten-free if you are sensitive to gluten)

Whole grain pastas made from artichoke, wheat, corn, quinoa, spelt, black beans, or rice

Vegetables and Fruits

Avocados, squashes, broccoli, kale, mustard greens, Swiss chard, cucumbers, carrots, radishes, dried figs, apples, plums, blood oranges, tomatoes, artichokes, cauliflower, brussels sprouts, eggplant, all kinds of mushrooms, salad greens, cherries, blueberries, limes, etc.

Vegetarian Cooking Stocks and Broths

Imagine Foods No Chicken Broth

Imagine Foods Vegetable Stock

Pacific Organic Mushroom Broth

Pacific Organic Vegetable Broth

Rapunzel Bouillon Cubes

Better Than Bouillon No Beef

Better Than Bouillon No Chicken

Nondairy

Cheeses: There are several companies whose products I use and enjoy. My favorite is Daiya, because it tastes and melts just like cheese. See www.daiyafoods.com.

Soya Kaas, Sunergia Soy Foods (www.sunergiasoyfoods.com);
Follow Your Heart (www.followyourheart.com); and Galaxy
Nutritional Foods (www.galaxyfoods.com) are all good, and
come in cheddar, mozzarella, Parmesan, and feta. Follow Your
Heart is what I use for eggplant Parmesan and hot paninis.

I like Silk Soy Creamer to mix into hot beverages. It's rich and
delicious.

Instead of cow's milk, try hemp, rice, almond, or soy milk.

Cream cheese and sour cream: Tofutti (www.tofutti.com)

Butter: Earth Balance Natural Buttery Spread. I use it in
everything that would call for butter, from baking and cooking to toast and muffins; it comes in sticks or tubs.

Pantry/Staples

Vegenaise mayonnaise substitute; use just like regular mayo,
but without the eggs (and better oil!).

Condiments: ketchup, mustard, relish. Annie's Naturals
are some of the best I've found (www.anniesnaturals.com).
Also, Cascadian Farm and Woodstock Farms are good
(www.cascadianfarm.com).

Canned goods: pasta sauces, beans, and vegetables. Try Eden
Organic (www.edenfoods.com); Muir Glen (www.muirglen.com);
Walnut Acres Organic (www.walnutacres.com). Good products.
I love Muir Glen Fire Roasted Diced Tomatoes!

Egg substitute: Ener-G Egg Replacer. It's nothing more than
potato starch and tapioca starch mixed into a powder, to which

you add water, and it works really beautifully for baking (www.ener-g.com).

In case you hadn't noticed, the best groceries are found fresh *on the periphery of the supermarket* or at your local farmers' markets. Try and choose colorful organic vegetables and fruits, and experiment with new foods you've never tried!

Cookbooks and Websites

Atlas, Nava. *Vegan Soups and Hearty Stews for All Seasons* (New York: Broadway, 2009).

Barnard, Tanya and Sarah Kramer. *How It All Vegan! 10th Anniversary Edition: Irresistible Recipes for an Animal-Free Diet* (Vancouver: Arsenal Pulp Press, 2009).

Freedman, Rory and Kim Barnouin. *Skinny Bitch in the Kitch* (Philadelphia: Running Press, 2007).

Gentry, Ann and Anthony Head. *The Real Food Daily Cookbook: Really Fresh, Really Good, Really Vegetarian* (New York: Ten Speed Press, 2005).

Geier, Catherine and Carol Brown. *Cafe Flora Cookbook* (San Francisco: HP Trade, 2005).

Klein, Donna. *Supermarket Vegan: 225 Meat-Free, Egg-Free, Dairy-Free Recipes for Real People in the Real World* (New York: Perigee Trade, 2010).

———. *Vegan Italiano: Meat-free, Egg-free, Dairy-free Dishes from Sun-Drenched Italy* (San Francisco: HP Trade, 2006).

Long, Linda. *Great Chefs Cook Vegan* (Hong Kong: Gibbs Smith, 2008).

Moskowitz, Isa Chandra and Terry Hope Romero. *Veganomicon: The Ultimate Vegan Cookbook* (Cambridge: Da Capo Lifelong Books, 2007).

Patrick-Goudreau, Colleen. *The Joy of Vegan Baking* (Beverly Hills: Fair Winds Press, 2007).

Peirson, Joy. *The Candle Cafe Cookbook: More Than 150 Enlightened Recipes from New York's Renowned Vegan Restaurant* (New York: Clarkson Potter, 2003).

Robertson, Robin. *Vegan Fire & Spice* (Woodstock, NY: Vegan Heritage Press, 2008); also *Quick Fix Vegetarian; 1000 Vegan Recipes; Vegan on the Cheap.*

Ronnen, Tal. *The Conscious Cook: Delicious Meatless Recipes That Will Change the Way You Eat* (New York: William Morrow Cookbooks, 2009).

Simpson, Alicia C. *Quick and Easy Vegan Comfort Food: 65 Everyday Meal Ideas for Breakfast, Lunch and Dinner with Over 150 Great-Tasting, Down-Home Recipes* (New York: The Experiment, 2009).

Wasserman, Debra and Charles Stahler. *Meatless Meals for Working People* (Baltimore: The Vegetarian Resource Group, 2004).

Recipe Websites

http://VegWeb.com

http://www.VeganCooking.com

http://VegCooking.com

http://www.ChooseVeg.com/vegan-recipes.asp

Health Websites

Dr. Neal Barnard, Physicians Committee for Responsible Medicine, www.pcrm.org

Dr. T. Colin Campbell, www.tcolincampbell.org

Dr. Caldwell Esselstyn, www.heartattackproof.com

Dr. Dean Ornish, www.pmri.org

Dr. John McDougall, www.drmcdougall.com

VegSource.com (for videos of all the above-mentioned doctors, blogs, articles, and more)

And for some good veganist info gathered into one place, visit me at www.kathyfreston.com!

Bon appétit!

ACKNOWLEDGEMENTS

WRITING THIS BOOK WAS PURE EXCITEMENT; EVERY DAY I WAS charged with adrenaline at the evidence, stories, and information that poured in to support the thesis that making a change in diet is a game changer. It was a symphony of contributions that I was lucky enough to weave together, and enormous thanks go to everyone who played a part:

My publishing team at Weinstein Books: Harvey Weinstein, Judy Hottensen, Kristin Powers, and Katie Finch—they are incredibly skillful at producing books, and I feel comfortably at home with them.

My new partners at Perseus: David Steinberger, Katie McHugh, and John Radziewicz who have been wonderful to work with.

Jennifer Rudolph Walsh, my agent at William Morris Endeavor, who has championed my ideas and helped me to run with them.

Emily Votruba, for her spot on copyediting, Ellen Rosenblatt for making the typesetting friendly, Brian

Chojnowski for the cover design, Charles Bush for his lovely cover photograph, and Nick Mullan who proofread and followed up on all the fact checking.

Bruce Friedrich, Chris Holbein, Stacy Davies, Margo Forker, Paula Moore, and Nicki Graham who each did research and/or answered my seemingly endless queries.

The doctors and nutritional scientists who shared with me their expertise and peer reviewed data: Dean Ornish, MD, T. Colin Campbell, PhD, Caldwell Esselstyn, MD, Neal Barnard, MD, and Michael Greger, MD.

Those who shared their stories and testimonials: Ben Goldsmith, Meg Wolff, Robert Dew, Natala Constantine, Ruth Heidrich, PhD, Bruce Wieland, Gene Baur, Josh Balk, Nathan Runkle (and his unnamed undercover investigator), and Philip Schein. And thanks to Rory Freedman, Joe Connelly, and Lisa Lange for making some of the connections.

The brilliant professor of theology and religious studies, Aaron Gross, without whom this book would not have the soulful substance it does. He schooled me, and provided much insight, academic research, and fascinating nuggets of religious history.

My beloved editor, Caroline Pincus, who artfully shaped and brought to life the manuscript; she is a literary midwife who has wisely and lovingly helped me with every word.

And finally, my husband Tom, who came up with the word Veganist, and who continues to be a gift and a blessing to me; I am forever grateful that we found our way to each other.